'There is so much here, so much tha‹  a strong sense that they are not alon their way through the maze (or ob most appropriate metaphor is). There is ⌐ professionals – to give them a better understanding of wₙₙ ₙ are going through, what they can do to help them, and some things that they should try to avoid. It is hard (probably impossible) for us to imagine what parents are going through – but there will be many, like myself, who will find that job significantly easier having read Stephanie's book, who will return to their work (once they have dried their eyes) with new ideas for how to be kind, how to empathise, how to help. The stories of all the people she has spoken to in the last year, all the families, and of course Daisy's stories, are the heart of the book. They speak volumes – bringing the children to life (and back to life). It is beautiful, moving and powerful.'

– *Prof Dominic Wilkinson, Consultant Neonatologist and Professor of Medical Ethics*

'Stephanie Nimmo has written a truly phenomenal book. *Anything for My Child* is both a lighthouse for any parent caring for a seriously ill child, as well as an instruction manual for any healthcare worker who cares for sick children and their families.'

– *Jared Rubenstein, MD, Paediatric Palliative Care Doctor*

'Steph Nimmo takes us on a journey few parents can ever be prepared for and helps us to understand, with clarity and compassion, why "doing anything" for a much-loved child might also mean letting them go.'

– *Sarah Barclay, Founder and Director, The Medical Mediation Foundation*

'From hospital to home, hospice and the courts, *Anything for My Child* transports the reader into the lives of families touched by the devastation of a terminal diagnosis. Essential reading, whether for professional or personal interest.'

– *Victoria Butler-Cole KC*

of related interest

Follow the Child
Planning and Having the Best End-of-Life Care for Your Child
Sacha Langton-Gilks
ISBN 978 1 78592 346 3
eISBN 978 1 78450 680 3

Bereaved Parents and their Continuing Bonds
Love after Death
Catherine Seigal
ISBN 978 1 78592 326 5
eISBN 978 1 78450 641 4

Love, Learning Disabilities and Pockets of Brilliance
How Practitioners Can Make a Difference to the
Lives of Children, Families and Adults
Sara Ryan
Forewords by Michael Edwards, Rob Mitchell and Elaine James
ISBN 978 1 78775 191 0
eISBN 978 1 78775 192 7

Anything for My Child

Making Impossible Decisions for Medically Complex Children

Stephanie Nimmo

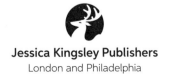

Jessica Kingsley Publishers
London and Philadelphia

First published in Great Britain in 2024 by Jessica Kingsley Publishers
An imprint of John Murray Press

1

A CIP catalogue record for this title is available from the
British Library and the Library of Congress

ISBN 978 1 80501 027 2
eISBN 978 1 80501 028 9

Printed and bound in Great Britain by TJ Books Ltd

Jessica Kingsley Publishers' policy is to use papers that are natural,
renewable and recyclable products and made from wood grown in
sustainable forests. The logging and manufacturing processes are expected
to conform to the environmental regulations of the country of origin.

Jessica Kingsley Publishers
Carmelite House
50 Victoria Embankment
London EC4Y 0DZ

www.jkp.com

John Murray Press
Part of Hodder & Stoughton Ltd
An Hachette Company

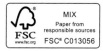

To Daisy Rose

You taught us all so much

'It was the touch of the imperfect upon the would-be perfect that gave the sweetness, because it was that which gave the humanity'

Thomas Hardy – *Tess of the D'Urbervilles*

Contents

Acknowledgements

THIS BOOK WOULD HAVE BEEN IMPOSSIBLE TO WRITE without the honesty and bravery of the people who freed up their time to tell me their stories. The parents: Nikki, Rosie, Sara, Gemma, Saira, Catherine, Sacha, Karina, Annette, Natalie, Catherine, Alan and Lucy, Dougal, Renata, Katie and all my online friends who responded to my random questions.

To Chloe (not forgetting the indomitable Isobel) and my own children who are still prepared to put up with their mum quizzing them about their childhood; thank you especially Xan for your honesty and insight.

To the nurses and doctors who knew Daisy and were part of our life, and especially those who shared their experiences of caring for my girl so openly and emotionally. To the paediatricians, intensivists and palliative consultants who taught me so much about what it's like to be in your shoes. To Ruth, for just getting it right from day one, the GPs and pharmacists who always did whatever they could to help us, and all the doctors and nurses that I met during Daisy's life or spoke to as part of my research.

To Dominic Wilkinson for the crash course in medical bioethics and the incredible insights you shared. And to all the ethicists, academics and professionals I spoke to as part of my research.

To Lisa for always being there on the end of the phone and putting up with my random messages when I needed to bounce an idea off someone medical.

To Romana and Nigel for helping me understand that the role of a chaplain transcends faith and beliefs.

To Esse and Sarah from the Medical Mediation Foundation for teaching me so much about mediation and communication.

To Hilary and all my colleagues at Together for Short Lives and The CoLab Partnership, thank you for all you do for children with medical complexity.

This book had some false starts; it's a difficult one for a publisher to take on and I'm grateful to Elen Griffiths at JKP for taking a punt on me!

To Simon for his proofing skills.

To Jan, for the admin support which ensured I could still pay my bills while working on this book.

To Finn for his questions about Daisy; you would have made her laugh!

To my darling children, Theo, Xanthe and Jules – it was never the childhood I wanted for you, but to watch you grow into incredible young people, despite everything life has thrown your way, gives me such joy. You will always be my greatest achievement, and I know your dad would have been so proud.

In loving memory of my brilliant friend, Lucy Watts MBE, and all the children and young people whose short lives taught us all so much: Daisy, DD, Lennon, Matthias, Livvy, Louie, Rhys, Oliver, Amy, Melody, Alicia, Ansley, Rocco, Charlie, Alfie, Alta, Archie, Jaymee, Danny – RIP.

Most of all, thank you, Calum. For so many things. This book is here because of your encouragement and support. Your feedback, questioning and journalistic tenacity to ensure I explored every angle was so essential. Thank you for the many evenings of conversation around so many topics that I was wrestling with, despite the fact you had your own work commitments and deadlines. Above all, thank you for being in my life and for showing me that life goes on.

Stephanie Nimmo
London, 2023

CHAPTER 1

The Crash Alarm

THE CRASH ALARM.

There's only one alarm in a hospital setting that's guaranteed to break through the alarm fatigue of constantly beeping medical devices. But, as a parent caring for a child who spends a lot of time in hospital, you soon get to know that sound – the searing, piercing scream that causes staff to drop what they are doing and run to its source. I don't know if it's the sound of the alarm per se or the response it elicits, but when the crash alarm goes off, you know it's serious.

I was in the parents' room when the crash alarm sounded for Daisy. In Great Ormond Street Hospital, that space is shared by both the paediatric (PICU) and neonatal (NICU) intensive care units. Parents from both wards sit, stony-faced, staring at phones, at the wall, talking in low voices, pacing. Every one of them grabbing a few welcome moments of respite over a cup of insipid coffee from the endless hours of waiting – sitting at their child's bedside, waiting for test results, updates from doctors, good news, bad news... watching monitors, hanging on every word, willing their child to improve...waiting.

Daisy's wheelchair was in the corner of the parents' room. It was piled high with all the paraphernalia you habitually collect as a parent caring for a child for whom the hospital was second home. Her favourite fleece blanket, an army of soft toys, books, pictures, the ubiquitous iPad...

Daisy had been transferred to PICU in the early hours of the morning, after the intensive care outreach team spent the night trying to stabilise her. I had heard the increasingly urgent negotiations for a bed to be made available in the PICU by the doctors trying to stabilise my child, phones ringing, discussions in low voices. Eventually, the call came, Daisy could not be stabilised and it was now time to move her to the intensive care ward. As I followed the nurses and doctors pushing Daisy's bed along the cold corridors at dawn, I wondered what had happened for a bed to be available. I knew that the ward had been full; it always was. These were the most specialist beds in the hospital. There had been murmurings of a specialist transfer to another hospital where an intensive care bed was available, but, in the end, this was not needed. Hopefully, a child had been well enough to be moved so that Daisy could have that bed. Or had a child died so that mine might have a chance to live?

It was lunchtime, and Daisy's breathing had been taken over by a ventilator. I was waiting in the parents' room while a physiotherapist performed a procedure called a bronchial lavage. I had been told it would help the doctors try to find out what bugs were in her lungs causing her body to shut down. I'd nodded my permission... I instinctively knew that we were beginning to lose the battle to stabilise my daughter. We always knew the enemy and how to manage it. She'd survived multiple episodes of sepsis; I could reel off the names of the bacteria that had been responsible as if they were ingredients in a recipe: *Pseudomonas*, Methicillin-resistant *Staphylococcus aureus*, *Candida*, *Klebsiella*, *Escherichia coli*...but it seemed that she was being attacked on all fronts. We had stared over the precipice many times, but this time felt different. This time, I knew we were going all the way.

I was attempting to distract myself by making a coffee, throwing some coins into the collection jar by the kettle to cover the cost of parent-room refreshments. I was sitting scrolling through my phone when the crash alarm sounded.

There were probably four other people plus me in the room at that moment – a young couple: she had long blonde hair, he had a dark beard; an older lady, maybe a child's grandma; another mother a bit younger than me – and we all rushed to the doorway. It seemed like everyone was rushing towards the PICU, I didn't need to be told where they were going. I knew.

'It's bed 16,' said the grandmother.

'That's my child,' I responded.

And with that, a nurse – the PICU family liaison nurse – swept me up, and together, we ran to Daisy's bed.

While the bronchial lavage was being performed, Daisy's heart had stopped, and the physiotherapist had pulled the crash alarm.

The next moments are seared into my brain. Here was my little girl – a few short weeks ago, we had celebrated her twelfth birthday, and then two days later she had torn off the wrapping paper of the new doll she had so desperately wanted for Christmas – like a ragdoll, bouncing on the bed as doctors performed CPR on her.

I couldn't watch. I held my head in my hands and cried out: 'It was not supposed to be like this.'

My voice came from a place I did not know. It was as though all the years of anguish and pain, the anticipation of this final moment, were all coming out. At every moment of Daisy's life, I had tried as much as possible to be calm and rational...to not fall apart in front of the teams caring for her, reserving my tears for the relative peace of an empty bathroom. But this felt wrong. This was not how she was supposed to die, with a doctor beating her chest back to life. This was not what I wanted for her. This was not how it was meant to be.

'She's back.' The nurse had been giving me a running commentary as the team worked on Daisy. These were the only words I could hear. I was aware that everyone had slipped away as quickly as they had arrived, and I was left, slumped in the plastic-covered chair, with the nurse by my side.

Daisy lay still again, tubes and lines covering her body, the beeps of the monitors and ventilator a familiar soundtrack. Finally, I knew what I had to do. I had been preparing for this all of her life.

'If she arrests again, I don't want her to be resuscitated,' I said. 'Let her go.'

I had lost count of the number of times I had been asked if my daughter was for 'full active resuscitation'. In other words, did I want her to be resuscitated in the event of a cardiac arrest? It was a standard question that we had to answer whenever she had a respite stay at the children's hospice that had supported us since Daisy was a baby. It was frequently asked when she was admitted into hospital. The answer was always yes.

Within a couple of short hours, as Daisy's organs shut down and her heart failed, I gave the nod to the intensivist hovering at my side and she switched off my daughter's ventilator. I had been given other options, all short-term fixes to buy us a little more time – dialysis, further resuscitation, more invasive procedures. But I knew that the most selfless thing I could do now for Daisy was the thing I wanted the least: I had to let her go. I had to let her die.

What had brought us to this point? After 12 years of caring for my youngest child – being her advocate, learning the procedures and regimens that would keep her alive, battling for her, sacrificing my career and ensuring that giving her a good quality of life was at the centre of my every waking moment – I was letting her die.

On the other side of the ward was the young couple who were also in the parents' room when the crash alarm had sounded. And just as I was preparing to remove my daughter's life support, they were preparing to launch a fight in the High Court to keep their son alive.

How do parents of the most medically complex children make decisions that no parent can ever contemplate making? What causes one family to want to try everything possible for their child, insist on leaving 'no stone unturned', while another is prepared to end life-supporting treatment as they feel it's in the best interests of their child?

Across the country...as many as three or four times every day, there are decisions made about life support for children or babies. Those decisions, in the vast majority of cases, are made jointly by families and health professionals. Parents or carers, together with the doctors and nurses looking after the child, come to a shared view that certain types of potentially life-prolonging treatment are not right for the child. That is not to say that these decisions are easy, or are made lightly. Quite the opposite: these are often agonising decisions, made only after much soul-searching, and after all other options have been considered and rejected. The point is rather that conflict and disagreement are not an inevitable or even a usual part of end-of-life decision-making for children. In many cases, in most cases, while decisions are difficult and distressing, they are able to be reached with the agreement of all those caring for the child – both professionals and family.[1]

What were the conversations that I had with professionals along my journey with Daisy that had brought me to this point, confident in knowing that I was doing the best thing for her (even if it didn't feel like the best thing for me)? Do all parents have similar conversations? Do they all feel as confident when their child reaches the end of life that they are making the right decision on behalf of their child?

And ultimately, when a parent talks about doing *anything for their child*, what does this mean? For some parents, it can mean mortgaging their home to take their child abroad for experimental treatment; for some, it can mean learning to manage a complex medical regimen to keep their child alive and at home; it can even mean being prepared to take on the emotional and financial toll of the family court to argue a case for continuing treatment. For me, it was many of those things and so much more. But in the end, anything for my child was to do the most selfless thing and let her go.

Over my years as Daisy's mum, I met many families, each caring for a child who was not expected to reach adulthood. Some, like Daisy, had been born that way, often as a result of a genetic disease; sometimes that disease was evident at birth, sometimes parents had taken home a seemingly healthy child only to witness deterioration

---

1   Wilkinson, D. and Savulescu, J. (2019) *Ethics, Conflict and Medical Treatment for Children: From Disagreement to Dissensus.* Elsevier Health Sciences, p.7.

and find themselves back in hospital months or even years later. Some children had an acquired condition – a catastrophic brain haemorrhage, cancer.

Every one of us had our own journey with our child, our own experience of being told our child would not reach adulthood, of good and bad communication with the professionals who were in place to support us and care for our child.

There are no right or wrong decisions when caring and advocating for a child who is not expected to reach adulthood. Only the most complex of ethical decisions. When I brought my first child home from the hospital and became a mother, I floundered. I was a successful professional, and yet the doctors and nurses in the busy London maternity hospital where I had given birth to my son only a few hours earlier had seen fit to discharge us home with no operating manual or user guide for this tiny life that depended on us for everything.

That feeling of helplessness is magnified a hundredfold when you care for a child who is medically complex and reliant on you to make the best decision possible. But that helplessness, in nearly every parent I have spoken to, soon turns into strength and determination to make the best possible decisions for their child.

Best possible decisions are also subjective decisions; there are so many influencing factors – demographics, age, experience, religious and cultural influences. Professionals have no control over these as they seek to work with families, but they have control over what they say to those families, how they say it and when...and these factors can influence the entire relationship.

I have learned that regardless of background or prior experience, there are still some common themes. Parents land into the world of caring for a medically complex child often with limited prior medical experience. They negotiate a huge learning curve to understand the language and jargon, and then to understand their own child's needs in order to be able to advocate on their behalf. Healthcare professionals are at an immediate advantage – they know how the system works, they've seen the scenarios before – and how they help parents navigate this new world can be crucial.

Regardless of the starting point, parents need to feel confident that their voices are heard, and professionals working with them have a role to play in helping them find their voice and be the best advocate for their child. I found that time and time again it boils down to a simple truth: taking time and listening without judgement.

Like many parents, I have been guilty of falling into a dynamic of combative language when describing my life with Daisy – life was a battle, for so many things – but that can set up conditions for conflict and mistrust. How can we move away from the language of combat to one of collaboration? How can parents and healthcare professionals build trust and understanding to work through disagreements so they do not become conflicts?

I don't have all the answers, but I explore these themes in the book, and by drawing on the lived experience of many other families, I illustrate how simple tipping points in communication and action can have long-lasting impacts.

Over the course of this book, you will get to know Daisy, learn about her life and also learn about the lives of other children and their parents. All of these families touched our life in some way. They are not strangers that became case studies for this book; they are all part of the web that is woven when a family finds themselves caring for a child who is not expected to reach adulthood.

In telling these stories, I am offering you all a glimpse into this world. All of us are one step away from it... I was once on the outside, but a sporadic and random gene mutation changed my world immeasurably.

I, like all the parents I met on my journey, was prepared to do anything for my child, but, as I learned, this can mean many things.

CHAPTER 2

Ordinary People, Extraordinary Circumstances

L IFE WASN'T ALWAYS LIKE THIS for any of us who care for children with medical complexity.

We all had a life before, a story that started before our arrival into the world of hospitals and monitors, drug regimens and difficult conversations.

We are all just ordinary people who have been catapulted – thanks to a gene mutation, a cancer diagnosis, a catastrophic event – into a new, alien world. Learning a new language and advocating for our child, judging what we feel is the best plan for them and our families. Deciding what, in our eyes, constitutes a good quality of life.

This could so easily be your story. None of us knows what's in the plan, how our life will unfold.

I was 36 when a late period and the familiar low-level nausea heralded the news that, once again, I was pregnant. This was a very much wanted and planned pregnancy for my husband Andy and me. Our fourth and last, the baby who would complete our family.

'According to our calculations, your baby has a one-in-four chance of having Down's syndrome.'

And, thinking back, that was when my life changed forever.

I don't remember the details. All I could hear was 'risk' and the words Down's syndrome and trisomy. I agreed to chorionic villus sampling (CVS) to take some cells from the placenta. This would definitely establish if the baby I was carrying did indeed have a chromosomal abnormality. It was not without risks, but it would give us information. There were two things I remember clearly about those conversations, however. First, we were immediately given the option of a termination if the test showed there was an abnormality, and that it was assumed that would be our plan. Second, we didn't understand that if the test was negative, that did not rule out our baby having some sort of genetic issue for which there was no test.

Shock clouds judgement. Maybe those things were explained, but all I took away was that there were two ways this could go – a termination or the all-clear.

The CVS was negative for Down's syndrome and other trisomies. We were told that I would need to go for a foetal echocardiogram when I was 20 weeks pregnant to rule out any cardiac defects.

Why would we need that? Weren't we in the clear for any problems?

I don't remember much about the foetal echocardiogram scan – just that it was OK and there didn't seem to be any problems with my baby's heart that they could detect. It was later with experience that I learned that just because something was not detectable, it didn't mean there wasn't a problem. I remember leaving feeling very reassured.

A couple of weeks later, however, things didn't seem to be right. I had always had small babies, but this baby seemed huge. Or rather my bump seemed huge. I was bursting out of my maternity clothes and becoming breathless with the pressure on my lungs.

I decided to drop into the antenatal clinic on my way home from work. The midwife on duty hadn't met me before, and she immediately assumed that I was full-term.

'Actually I'm 24 weeks pregnant,' I told her.

'You are measuring very big for your dates,' she replied. 'I think we need to scan you.'

I had polyhydramnios.[1] Too much amniotic fluid. I was off the scale.

Hindsight is a wonderful thing. I now know that severe poly-hydramnios is an indicator that things are not right with the devel-oping baby, but again I just heard the words 'everything is within normal limits' when the obstetrician looked at the measurements of my developing baby.

Things seemed to happen pretty quickly then. I was told that the increased fluid put me at greater risk of premature birth. I was given steroid injections to help the baby's lungs mature, and amniotic fluid was drawn out of my ever-growing belly every few days. I began to get used to the big syringes plunging into my tight-as-a-drum stomach, drawing out pints of pale-pink fluid. I lay in my hospital bed that night hoping that the procedure didn't send me into premature labour, willing my child to hang on in there a little longer.

I couldn't eat. The pressure of my huge bump pressed against my stomach so that every mouthful felt like a full meal. I began to itch unbearably as bile acid built up in my body, and I was exhausted both from the toll this pregnancy was taking and the anaemia that I had developed.

Back at home, Andy was trying to keep things going with the help of our childminder and our close network of friends. Christmas was coming, and our children were easily distracted by school plays and Christmas parties.

'I've spoken to the neonatal consultant, and we have agreed that your baby needs to be delivered,' the obstetrician told me.

I'd reached 33 weeks in my pregnancy.

On the morning of 22nd December 2004, I was taken into an operating theatre. It had been decided that it was going to be safer for me and my baby if she was delivered by caesarean section. There was so much amniotic fluid and I was so exhausted that it was deemed too risky to attempt a vaginal birth. I was relieved. It

---

1   NHS (2020) 'Polyhydramnios (too much amniotic fluid).' www.nhs.uk/
conditions/polyhydramnios

ANYTHING FOR MY CHILD

was time this baby came out. I didn't care that it was just before Christmas and she would go straight to NICU (neonatal intensive care unit) after delivery.

Daisy Rose was dragged into the world at 9.30 a.m. on Wednesday 22nd December 2004. She was blue and angry and puffed up full of fluid. I was allowed a brief moment to touch her face before she was whisked away to be stabilised.

I got to see her a few hours later. She seemed so much bigger than the other babies in their incubators, not surprising given how much water she had been floating around in over the last few weeks. She was attached to a continuous positive airway pressure (CPAP) machine, forcing oxygen into her lungs, pushing her nose up. There seemed to be tubes and monitors everywhere. Alarms beeped and pinged. Years later, I would be able to name all of those tubes, machines and alarms, and I would learn how to set them up, but for now, this was an alien world to me.

I looked at my new baby in her plastic box. A nurse opened a window in the side of it and I reached in my hand and touched the tiny little cheek. 'Hello, Daisy Rose.'

This was my introduction to my new life. A life a million miles away from anything I'd known so far.

Nothing in my previous life prepared me for this new world experience of hospitals; my last child had been born at home and, apart from two other births and a couple of minor surgeries, I'd managed to avoid them.

The language, life and culture of hospitals were an enigma to me.

I didn't know how the hierarchies of doctors worked, who did what in hospitals, the daily rituals of ward rounds, handovers, lunch breaks, named nurses. It was a new and alien world.

It was also very clear that I was not just passing through. From the moment Daisy arrived in NICU, the doctors were concerned that prematurity was the least of her worries. The first words that Andy heard when he was called to see his new daughter once she had been stabilised were, 'We think she may have a form of dwarfism'.

I was numb and exhausted, I'd just been through major surgery,

I had postnatal hormones coursing through my body, I was desperately trying to express breast milk, I was separated from my other children, and it was Christmas time.

By Christmas Day, Daisy's care had been stepped down from the intensive care room to high dependency. Her breathing was more stable, and she needed less intervention. I would learn to appreciate these milestones over the years, but for now it was just all so new and I hung on every word the doctors and nurses said.

It was clear to me that I was going to have to become very familiar with this new world. This little girl needed me, not just to be her mum, but I would need to be her advocate, her voice. I would need to learn how this system worked in order to speak on her behalf, in order to give her the best chance.

The prospect was overwhelming. I felt disempowered, in a strange country, where everyone was looking at me and our lives were no longer our own.

Like living in a goldfish bowl. I hear this from parents over and over, that once they are the parent of a child with complex needs, their lives are on display. I would sit in the neonatal unit and watch nurses writing up Daisy's notes, wondering what they were saying. My ears would burn when staff arrived for handover. I knew they weren't just talking about Daisy – they seemed to know far too much about the rest of my family. I soon realised that no information I shared in conversation was kept private.

'How's your husband coping?' I remember one nurse asking. We were in an ambulance taking Daisy for a detailed heart scan at a specialist hospital. 'He must be finding it hard with his depression.'

How did she know Andy had depression? (He'd been on treatment for it for a few years; it wasn't something we were ashamed of, but it was also something that, at that stage, we had not talked about much in public.) The realisation hit me that we were the subject of conversation in the staff room – every emotional outburst, non-appearance of Andy on the ward, hints that I was struggling. I felt as if I was on display, the life of my family on view. What were they writing about us? What were they saying?

When you learn your child has some sort of extra going on – a life-limiting condition, complex medical needs, a sudden life-changing diagnosis – your life is no longer your own. When Daisy arrived, I felt that our whole life, our family, was viewed by people who only had a small snapshot of it. Very few people took the time to get to know us as people, and those who did were the ones who stayed the course. Because, despite it all, despite the feelings of intrusion, I instinctively knew that we had to build our team. There was no way I could do this on my own.

Not every child who is diagnosed with a life-limiting condition starts their life in the neonatal unit: some go home after a seemingly normal pregnancy and birth only to fail developmental milestones; some children are healthy and then acquire a condition that renders them life-limited.

This is my story, but I didn't want this to be just my story, my personal experience of life with Daisy. I wanted to know if it was something about me, my prior experience and background, that had shaped the communications and decisions that were made about my child or whether there were some common themes that everyone experienced.

I have spoken to many families, not just during my time researching this book but over the years caring for Daisy. This has helped me maintain a degree of objectivity as I explore some of my own experiences.

Over the years since Daisy's birth, I crossed paths with many other families. Every one of us has our own unique story to tell, all united as exclusive members of a club caring for a medically complex child. Some of us are in the club that no one wants to join: bereaved parents, the parents with empty arms.

Nikki is one of those parents. We knew each other from membership of various special needs parenting forums as well as bumping into each other during outpatient appointments at Great Ormond Street Hospital.

Nikki's story

Nikki's first-born child was a son called Lennon. He too arrived in the world via the neonatal unit. She had only been dating Ian, Lennon's father, for a few months, but they decided to make a go of it, buying a flat and preparing for life as a family of three.

Things were progressing well with her pregnancy until Nikki's blood pressure began to rise dangerously high and her puffy ankles signified retained water. As debilitating headaches developed, it was clear that Nikki had developed pre-eclampsia, a very serious antenatal condition that could threaten both her life and her unborn baby's life if left unchecked. Nikki was admitted into hospital and, like me, given the steroid shot to help her unborn baby's lungs develop. All her baby scans had been fine; the biggest worry was Nikki's health and how long doctors could keep her safe so that her unborn baby could have the best chance possible.

Then a scan showed that her baby's umbilical cord wrapped around his neck and he was in distress.

'The consultant literally threw a set of scrubs at my partner and told him to put them on as they were taking me to theatre immediately,' said Nikki.

As Nikki was being prepared for an emergency caesarean section, a nurse arrived from the hospital neonatal unit. She explained to Nikki that her baby would be very small because he was only 28 weeks' gestation and he might need to go on to a ventilator for breathing support.

'You'll probably only be in the neonatal unit for about eight to ten weeks,' the nurse told Nikki. 'Just until your baby's lungs are strong enough for him to go home.'

'Oh, if I knew then what I know now,' Nikki told me. 'Six months later, we got to take our baby home, and not for very long...'

She had a brief look at her newborn son before he was whisked away to the neonatal unit where he was put on a ventilator. The next day, 24 hours after delivering him, Nikki was wheeled down to the unit to have a first proper glimpse of her baby through a window.

'He's not doing as well as expected,' the nurse caring for Lennon told Nikki.

Nikki returned to her bed on the antenatal ward, in pain and bleeding heavily, listening to the sound of newborn babies outside, not knowing what was happening with her son.

'It was all just surreal,' she told me. 'And I didn't say anything because I just thought, well, I don't want to make a fuss – they're all busy.'

Two days after Lennon was born, the neonatal consultant spoke to Nikki and her partner, Ian. He told them that Lennon had developed a bleed in his lungs and needed to be moved to another hospital to be put on an oscillating ventilator.

The specialist transfer team was called, and it took eight hours to stabilise Lennon enough to be transferred to the new hospital safely. Once the specialist intensive care ambulance left, the realisation hit Nikki that she might never see her son alive again.

She begged to be allowed to follow the ambulance, but the nursing staff refused: she was too sick herself, and they could not spare a staff member to accompany her.

'It was just not fair,' Nikki recalled. 'My child, whom I had barely seen but had carried inside me, was dying on his own in a hospital miles away, and I couldn't be there. No one was updating me – we literally did not know if he was dead or alive, or what was happening. It was just horrendous.'

Eventually, when she was able to see Lennon, she was told that his life was still in the balance, that things were very much touch and go.

And if all of this wasn't enough, Nikki's health began to deteriorate. She started having seizures and was readmitted to the hospital. She was eventually stabilised but was clearly too unwell to leave the hospital to be at Lennon's side, and her partner, Ian, was torn. He wanted to be with his sick baby, but he also did not want to leave Nikki's side.

So often in the stories of children with complex needs, it's the action of one person that can make a difference – the tipping point that can make or break a situation. It just takes one person to take ownership, whether or not it's in their job description, to make a huge difference for a family. I've heard stories of doctors sorting out emergency prescriptions so that families can go away on a much-needed holiday, making calls on their days off, making home visits, just going above and beyond.

That's what Ruth did for us. Ruth was the attending consultant for the neonatal unit on the day that Daisy was born. It meant that Daisy became her patient. Ruth was not long back from maternity leave herself, and it soon transpired that she had grown up in the area where Andy and I lived. In another world, I like to think that Ruth would be one of my mum friends, the sort you chat to at the school gate and meet up with at book clubs and girls' nights out. She was the person who I could rely on to just 'get it'. And, later, Daisy's palliative consultant and even our GP – these were the people who could write letters, make calls, turn around prescriptions so that we could get on and have some semblance of family life. Much of what they did was not in their main job description, but their actions made all the difference, even though it was probably an additional burden of responsibility for them.

And this is what happened with Nikki. The ward sister where she was now an inpatient recognised her as one of her daughter's schoolfriends. Now Nikki was no longer 'just another patient'. There was a human connection, A bed for Nikki was found in the same hospital as Lennon and at least Nikki could be nearby.

Lennon was a very poorly baby. It was becoming evident that this was not solely due to his prematurity. 'No one was asking the question, "Why is this child behaving in this way?"' Nikki said. 'No one was trying to join up the dots and look at the big picture here.'

'You know how they leave the x-ray films up on screens after viewing them?' Nikki told me. 'I remember one doctor saying we needed to talk, and as she took Ian and me into her office, she waved at the screen which had an x-ray of Lennon's lungs and said, "This is all white and it should be black."' Nikki was left confused. She wanted to ask more questions, she wanted details, to know why this was happening, but no one was talking to her; it felt as if she was just an extra, not the mother of the child in question.

'It really felt like we lurched from crisis to crisis in those neonatal days,' Nikki told me. 'Firefighting, just to get Lennon to the point where he was stable enough to be at home. We felt that was the endpoint. We were too inexperienced and naive to ask why no one was focused on what was causing all of these setbacks.'

After six long and eventful months, Lennon came home. He still needed oxygen and very close monitoring. The joy of bringing their son home at last was short-lived. Within weeks, he was back in hospital again. And so his story continued, just like Daisy, and like so many complex children where prematurity is not the main cause of their problems, bouncing in and out of hospital as his stressed and tired parents tried to make a life, tried to find answers, tried to find some sort of normal existence in this new and unpredictable world.

I was fortunate. From very early on, it was clear that Daisy's main issues were not down just to her prematurity. We had a neonatal consultant who was determined to find answers and, unlike Nikki's early experience, she didn't make getting Daisy home the endgame.

Early Tipping Points

'STEPH, I DON'T KNOW WHAT'S GOING ON WITH DAISY, but we'll work together to find the answers.'

Over my time as Daisy's mum, there were many tipping points that set the tone for my interactions with healthcare professionals. Some are good, and some are not so good. This early meeting with Ruth was a crucial tipping point. She was that personal connection that took us from just another patient to Daisy and her family. We were very fortunate that we found someone we could trust early on, who showed by her actions and not just her words that she was on our side.

Daisy had been in the neonatal unit for about ten days when I first met Ruth. Daisy had progressed from the intensive care area through to high dependency, and now she was in the special care unit. This was the last stop before home. The babies no longer needed breathing support or too much intervention and were mainly being stabilised on feed regimens to gain weight.

While Daisy's breathing hadn't been a significant cause for concern at that point, feeding was a massive issue. Daisy was failing to thrive. She was out of the incubator and now in a plastic cot, and the last tube that remained was the one from her nose into her stomach. Every day, I would wait for my turn to take my place in the curtained alcove where the breast pump sat, and I attempted to pump enough milk to last for the next 24 hours.

A feeding schedule was in place to try to get Daisy to take

increased volumes of expressed breast milk to give her nutrition and keep her hydrated. Every few hours, a syringe of my precious milk was poured into the tube in Daisy's nose, into her stomach. As I poured the milk into the syringe, Daisy screamed and screamed. Her stomach was distended, and she arched her back. The one thing that I needed to be able to do as Daisy's mum, to give her nutrition, seemed to cause her pain and distress. It was traumatic for both of us.

One day, Ruth came to see me in the special care unit and asked me if I could join her to chat about Daisy. I willingly agreed. I felt we were going nowhere fast. Daisy seemed to be constantly unsettled and crying, she barely slept, and I couldn't even think about how I would manage at home without the support of the nursing staff.

Ruth made me a coffee, and I followed her into the cramped doctor's office. Clutching the mug, she pulled up a chair for me and shut the door. It was a relief not to hear the constant hum of the neonatal unit, to be out of that busy environment – the beeping monitors, clattering of trolleys, crying babies, crying parents, the crashing lids of the yellow metal clinical waste bins.

'Is there anything unusual that you have noticed about Daisy?' asked Ruth.

After nearly two weeks on the ward, getting to know my new daughter, I could see that there was something not right. This was definitely more than just prematurity.

But 'Um, I don't know...she really arches her head back when she's in the cot' was all that I could offer in response.

I just didn't know. She was so different from my other children. None of them had been premature, so in many ways, I felt like a first-time parent. I couldn't put my finger on it; I was just happy that Daisy had progressed through the various stages of the unit. Only a few weeks before, I had been struggling with a very diffi-cult pregnancy; I'd had a caesarean delivery; I'd spent Christmas in hospital, separated from my other children, trying to express milk for my new baby.

I'd faced the trauma of leaving the maternity unit without my baby, travelling to the hospital every day to be with her. In addition, my husband was experiencing a relapse of his depression. To cap it all, I had developed an infection in my uterus and needed to start a course of antibiotics.

I was tired, zombie-tired, full of postnatal hormones, but I had to engage my brain. I had to hold it all together because, clearly, there was something going on with my new baby.

'We've noticed a few things,' continued Ruth. 'Her cry is very weak, for example, but she also is very unsettled.'

Oh yes, she was. She cried a lot. In fact, sometimes the night staff had to wheel her little plastic cot out of the main ward and put her next to the nurses' station as she cried so much that she was waking the other babies, weak cry and all.

'I would like to run some tests,' said Ruth. 'That way, we can rule things out, hopefully, and start to get closer to finding out what's going on with Daisy. I think it would be a good idea for a geneticist to come and take a look at her too, if that's OK with you?' she continued.

Of course, it was OK with me. I trusted Ruth, I had immediately warmed to her, and I knew that we needed to get to the bottom of what was going on with Daisy so that I could begin to understand what she needed from me and how I could help her.

I was trying to avoid searching online for answers and I could barely think about what was going to happen the next day, let alone the next weeks, or months or even years of life with Daisy. I felt safe putting my trust in Ruth, and she didn't overwhelm me with complex medical terms or scare me with possible scenarios. In that room, I just felt that she was an empathetic human being who understood what I was going through and was prepared to try to help.

As we were finishing our conversation, she asked me one last question. It was another really important tipping point in my journey with Daisy.

'Who's your favourite GP, Steph?'

We all have a favourite GP – the one that we try to get an

appointment with, the one that we know will go that extra mile. In our local practice, it was Dr Mason. So I gave her that name.

'If it's OK with you, I'm going to call him regularly while Daisy is here. You are going to need a good relationship with your GP when you get home with Daisy, and it's important he's up to speed and knows what's going on so that he can sort things out quickly if you need him to.'

And for the eight weeks that Daisy was in the neonatal unit, Dr Mason had regular phone updates from Ruth about what was happening. She was right: I needed our community services more than ever once I became Daisy's mum, and for all those years I cared for Daisy, I just needed to call and our GP practice would sort out whatever I needed.

This is how joined-up communication between healthcare professionals happens. Thinking about who needs to be involved in the patient's life, how they are going to cope at home. Not just banging out a discharge letter and cc'ing lots of people, but thinking about the people who would be able to help support the family and keeping them in the loop. Establishing communication links and picking up the phone, or even just writing a quick email – it could make a world of difference to a family who needs to feel that they are supported and that the people who are there to support them know what is going on.

The tests that Ruth had ordered began that day, as we tried to understand what was going on with this little girl who hadn't even hit her due date yet. She had armfuls of blood taken, and she even took her first trip out of the unit as I wheeled her along the cold hospital corridors to have x-rays and ultrasounds.

I had been trying to persist with breastfeeding to top up Daisy's milk, but one of the tests showed that while she could suck, she was in danger of aspirating milk into her lungs, increasing her risk of chest infections. It looked as though that tube in her nose was going to have to stay a little longer. However, none of the scans of her stomach gave us any clue as to why feeding was causing so much pain and distress.

I was sitting by Daisy's cot when I saw the genetics consultant arrive at the nurses' station and ask for Daisy's notes. I really did not know what a geneticist was supposed to do. I thought we had established that there was nothing wrong genetically with Daisy following the antenatal testing, but from the sound of it, this was not the case. I really had not understood that antenatal testing was limited, that a negative test for Down's did not mean that Daisy didn't have some sort of genetic issue.

The doctor pulled up a chair and sat next to Daisy's cot. She asked if she could examine her, and I nodded my permission.

She picked Daisy up and described her in medical terms I did not recognise: epicanthal folds, low-set ears, flattened nasal bridge... what was this all about? She was describing dysmorphic features that indicated that there was some sort of genetic abnormality.

Dysmorphic features. That was the first time I heard that term. I felt that she was telling me my little girl, my newborn daughter, my Daisy, was ugly.

'There is a lot of research taking place at the moment into genetic conditions that are caused by changes in genes in a very specific cellular pathway,' the geneticist explained. 'We haven't found out what that change or mutation is, but we think that it's common in a group of syndromes that all have very similar presentations but different degrees of severity.'

She went on to tell me that one of the syndromes caused by this mutation was called Costello syndrome, that there was no genetic test for the syndrome at that time and the diagnosis was made by clinical presentation over the course of the child's early years.

'We'll have to wait and see,' she continued. 'Hopefully, it's not that one, though, because it's the most severe of the syndromes of the gene pathway.'

I looked at her, barely able to take it all in. She told me she would send me some information, and with that, she went to scribble in Daisy's notes and was gone.

I was left, alone, on the busy ward. Just as my first meeting with

Ruth had been a positive tipping point in communications, this first encounter with the geneticist was a negative one.

It hadn't even occurred to me that this information should have been given to me away from the ward, and with the opportunity for my husband, or at least a friend, to be present. Ruth's request to be paged so she could attend the meeting had been ignored. I'd been given some earth-shattering news about my child in an open ward, in full hearing of everyone else, and then left on my own to take it all in.

Asking to move away from the open ward or to have someone else with me during the conversation with the geneticist did not feel like something in my power. She seemed rushed, as if Daisy was another item on her 'to do' list for the day. Yet this woman was giving me information that would change my life forever.

The promised information about this potential syndrome never did arrive, and that night I found myself firing up Google and reading terrifying information about the increased risk of malignancy, serious heart problems, bone issues and learning disability.

Did my girl have this awful disease? Was I really going to have to watch and wait to see if all these awful things happened to her to have a confirmed diagnosis?

Daisy came home just after her due date, eight weeks after her delivery. Over those weeks, I had watched the season change as leaves began to open up on the tree outside the neonatal unit. Finally, spring was coming, and we would have all our family under one roof.

Our other three children were beside themselves with excitement as we brought Daisy into the house. They didn't see dysmorphic features; they just saw their baby sister.

Coming home, however, was just the start.

Daisy didn't settle. She cried all night, and I worked and worked to get enough milk into her. She arched her back and just did not seem comfortable, no matter how much we tried to rock and soothe her.

We tried to have some sort of routine, but we were already

running on empty. Andy was back at work, and I was relying on friends to take my other children to school and the childminder.

Letters started dropping through the door – brown envelopes 'for the parent or guardian of Daisy Nimmo', appointments for the services that were starting to fall into place. A review with a community paediatrician, follow-up appointments with Ruth, with the paediatric dietitian...

The health visitor came to see us, and I held up Daisy's dry nappy. 'I just can't get enough fluid into her,' I wailed. She promised to come back and keep an eye on things.

But we were becoming increasingly anxious. Daisy began to have odd flushing episodes. Her cheeks burning red, she cried out in pain and arched her back. We were experienced parents, but we did not know what was wrong with our daughter.

We were at our wits' end, and so, only a few weeks after we had brought Daisy home from the hospital, we found ourselves in the paediatric accident and emergency department, desperately worried that something very serious was going on with our little girl.

The doctor on duty that evening had been one of the regular doctors in the neonatal unit; it was a relief to see someone who already knew our daughter.

'We couldn't keep you in the neonatal unit indefinitely, but it was clear that something was happening with Daisy; that's why we were almost waiting for that crisis,' he explained.

I've never forgotten those words. I wish I'd known that the team in the neonatal unit had been feeling like that, that something was about to happen. I remember there was a lot of head scratching and deep sighs, but I wish more of them had said, 'We don't know what's going on with Daisy' – just as Ruth had.

At times, I felt that some of the doctors were clutching at straws, wanting to give me an answer, almost as if they wanted to be the one to make the big breakthrough, to work out why Daisy was failing to thrive and her feeding causing so many issues. I just needed to know that when we went home with Daisy, they weren't giving up on us. I needed to know what they didn't know. I just needed to

ANYTHING FOR MY CHILD

know that people were with us, trying to find out why Daisy was the way she was.

Many of the tests that Ruth had originally ordered could take a while to be processed – they needed to be sent to specialist labs, and time had to elapse to establish a result – so we didn't have all the information we needed, and sometimes that can take many months.

One of the specialist tests had come back, however. It showed that Daisy had something called raised catecholamine levels. Catecholamines are hormones that are released into the blood when a person is under physical or emotional stress. Consistently raised levels can also indicate the presence of a rare cancerous tumour.

Did this explain her flushing episodes and pain? I felt a mixture of terror and relief. I needed to know what we were dealing with – but a cancer diagnosis? Daisy was only a couple of months past her due date, tiny and vulnerable. How the hell was she going to be able to get through this?

Suddenly, there seemed to be a focus, and frantic calls were made between the doctors at our local hospital and specialist cancer centres. Within a couple of days, we found ourselves in another new alien world. This was the world of specialist care – a step up from the district general hospital. Daisy was now on an oncology ward at Great Ormond Street Hospital. Its reputation went before it as a centre of excellence in paediatric medicine and research.

I remember feeling a huge sense of relief. These people will have the answers, they will sort Daisy out, and then we can get back on with being a family again.

It seems so naive in hindsight, knowing what I know now, but I was an amateur in those days. I was learning how the system worked and just how far medical science was able to help. I truly believed at that time that the doctors caring for Daisy would have all the answers, yet over the months and years, I learned that we as a society have been lulled into a false sense of security. We hear about breakthroughs, new treatments, cures – the media focuses on the successes, the good news stories, the cures, the children who live.

Stories about children dying, children who can't be helped, these don't make good press. Nobody wants to hear about what medical science cannot do, only what it can.

'When we reach this point of complexity, it's really just academic guesswork,' a junior doctor once told me. He was right. It was a real wake-up call for me, as it is for so many parents of children who are caring and advocating for a child who is medically complex. We expect doctors who treat our children to have all the answers, to know what to do, to make things better. What happens if they can't? Where do we go then?

CHAPTER 4

How Do You Do It?

WITHIN A FEW SHORT MONTHS, my life had changed beyond measure. I was mourning the child I thought I was going to have while learning to love this new baby who needed me in ways so much more complex and extreme than my other children.

I was fighting guilt about the impact on the lives of my other children, aged seven, five and two. They had just experienced a Christmas without their mother, without their new sister. My younger son, Jules, had been born at home, in a birth pool. When my older two woke up on that warm August morning, they met their new brother, pink and perfect, in his Moses basket next to my bed. Now, their first experience of Daisy was to peer through a plastic box while a nurse explained what all the machines she was connected to were for.

I had gone from leading a team at a busy college, reassuring my boss that I would return from maternity leave in order to make sure everything was ready for our busiest time of the year, student enrolment in the following September, to feeling as if I was a child again, surrounded by adults speaking in a different language.

I felt compliant in the hands of the medical professionals who were caring for my child. But a realisation soon began to dawn when the answers didn't come, when doctors contradicted themselves or each other, when they struggled to tell me what they thought was going on with Daisy. At some point, the penny dropped: it was down to me; I had to be the one to speak for

Daisy, to notice all the little things, to ask the questions, to push for answers.

People who meet me think I'm an extrovert, that I'm confident and self-assured. That's the impression I give, but, deep down, I am riddled with self-doubt and imposter syndrome. So when Daisy arrived into my life, I had to get over all of that, draw from my professional experience, pull down the emotional shutters and be the person that Daisy needed me to be so that we could all get through this.

I was an experienced mum, but I felt like a first-time mother all over again.

In my research for this book, I have spoken to many parents. I wanted to discover if the feelings and experiences I had would have been different if I had been, for example, a first-time mother or discovered later in my child's life that there was a problem after a seemingly normal birth and early-years journey.

Every single parent I spoke to told me that they had felt disempowered and voiceless in the early days. But each had found that regardless of any prior life experience, they would need to become their child's voice and advocate. Time after time, parents told me of experiencing a transition from passive compliance to a realisation that doctors did not have all the answers for their child.

There are always clear tipping points in a parent's journey – good examples where they felt empowered to work with doctors and ask probing questions, and negative examples where disagreements may allow disputes and conflicts to arise.

When Ruth invited me into her office, and we drank coffee together as she told me that she didn't know what was going on with my daughter, that became a tipping point in how I saw doctors. They are humans, trying to use their knowledge to help. For me, this was the point where I actually felt reassured: I could feel Ruth's empathy with my situation and that she really did want to try to work out what was going on so that we could work out what Daisy needed from all of us.

Gemma's story

Gemma had learned at her 20-week scan that there was a problem with her pregnancy.

She had instinctively known that something was not right. '"Oh, it's just first-time mum nerves," people kept saying,' she told me. '"And the fact that you know too much because of your job, you just think things are going wrong." But I knew that it was more than this.'

Gemma is a paediatric nurse with extensive experience in caring for children with life-limiting and terminal conditions. I first met her at Shooting Star Children's Hospice in Guildford when she was Daisy's named nurse.

I was keen to speak to Gemma because I wanted to understand if having a background in paediatric care had made her feel more empowered, almost giving her a head start when things didn't go according to plan in her first pregnancy.

'I went for my ultrasound scan,' Gemma told me, 'and I was really nervous, and I told the radiographer that I worked in a children's hospice and that I was worried something was wrong. She told me not to worry, that I knew too much, that everything would be fine.'

But it wasn't. By that afternoon, Gemma was being scanned in a specialist foetal medicine clinic in central London.

'The nurse began to tell me what was wrong with the baby's heart, and I stopped her and said, "I know, it's tetralogy of Fallot",' Gemma recalls.

Tetralogy of Fallot is a rare congenital condition where four abnormalities occur in the heart. Decades ago, it was fatal, but thanks to antenatal screening and advanced surgical techniques, a child born with the syndrome has a far better chance of survival.

Gemma agreed to have an amniocentesis test that day in order to rule out any other genetic factor, and the possibility of a late termination was discussed with her as she signed the consent forms.

Gemma was really frank when she confessed to me that she knew she could cope with a baby with complex medical needs, but one that had learning disabilities, a developmental delay – that was another thing. I'd felt exactly the same. My first instinct when I'd been told that I had a one-in-four chance of having a child with Down's was that I would not be able to cope with a child with a learning disability.

Daisy did have a learning disability, and learning how to care for her and how to understand her needs taught me a lot. Life with Daisy showed me that experience is always the best teacher.

Gemma's amniocentesis didn't show any other problems with her baby, and she proceeded with the pregnancy knowing that her daughter would probably require several surgeries at a very young age. Gemma had nursed children with the same condition and knew that, thanks to advances in medical science and surgical techniques, the outlook for children born with tetralogy of Fallot was very good.

Gemma's daughter, Zoe, was born at nearly full-term. After two weeks in the neonatal unit, the doctors decided that she could go home, and plans were made for her to return at a later date for her first heart surgery.

Gemma's experience as a nurse meant that she understood the implication of what was happening a lot more quickly than less experienced parents. Despite her medical training and experience, however, she still felt disempowered. She was a new mum now, not a nurse, and life on the other side of the hospital bed was proving very difficult.

Like many newborns, Zoe was yellow with jaundice, but when, after a few weeks at home and regular exposure to daylight, the jaundice did not improve, Gemma began to worry. She mentioned her concerns at a developmental review appointment with her community health visitor.

'She told me not to worry,' Gemma said. 'She told me that I was overthinking.'

But Gemma's instinct was right. A few days later, Gemma took Zoe for an outpatient check-up with her hospital consultant. He was immediately very concerned at how jaundiced she appeared.

'I was cross with myself for listening to the health visitor,' Gemma recalled. 'I knew something wasn't right, I knew the signs,

I'm a nurse, but the health visitor made me feel that I was just an over-anxious first-time mother.'

That experience has lived with Gemma. Chatting to her, there were some familiar themes: she was full of postnatal hormones, she was caring for a child with a serious heart defect who would soon need major surgery, but even though she was an experienced nurse, she still felt disempowered and let down by people who should have listened to her, taken her concerns seriously.

Gemma was right to be concerned because it soon turned out that there was more to Zoe than tetralogy of Fallot. Zoe did not have normal newborn jaundice; she had a rare genetic disease that was affecting both her liver and her heart – a disease so rare it would not have been picked up in an amniocentesis test.

Unfortunately, Gemma would learn that her daughter had a confirmed diagnosis of Alagille syndrome almost as an aside from a registrar as he checked Zoe's notes, during a routine phone call to the hospital to order medication.

And so, instead of being taken into a room with her partner and told the news, instead of being given the opportunity to ask questions and understand the implications of this bombshell for their daughter, Gemma was alone, at home with only the internet to turn to as she sought to understand what this diagnosis meant for her child.

Doctors and nurses tell me the theory, how it's supposed to be done: take both parents aside, make sure you have time and are not rushed, make sure you give them time and space, speak to them in a quiet room off the ward, let them ask questions, give them any information they need.

Gemma learned about her daughter's life-limiting diagnosis because someone had written the test results into her daughter's notes communicating the plan for how the parents would be informed of the news. It meant that the registrar who spoke to Gemma when she phoned the hospital to arrange a prescription really had no idea of the impact of his throwaway comment.

Alagille syndrome is a rare, life-limiting condition. In some

ANYTHING FOR MY CHILD

cases, a liver transplant can be an option. Zoe experienced multiple health setbacks, and after several white-knuckle journeys in intensive care, Gemma and her partner were eventually told that Zoe would not be a candidate for a transplanted liver as her heart condition was too complex and severe for that surgery to be a viable or even survivable option.

'We were told the news by the intensive care consultant,' Gemma told me. 'The liver team were pushing for a transplant, but the cardiac team decided that Zoe's heart would not be able to undergo the surgery. They discussed a multiple heart, lung and liver transplant, but finally, it was decided that none of these would be an option.' At that point, they were introduced to the palliative care team.

'That's where my experience as a nurse was really beneficial,' she explained. 'I already knew what we were facing before the consultant mentioned it, and I quickly accepted the support from the palliative team; even though Zoe was not at the end of life, nor likely to be for a long time, I knew that it would be good have them in our lives. In fact, I'd already asked for a referral to a children's hospice because I understood the help they could offer me. I was a first-time mum, and all the other mums I'd met at antenatal group had healthy babies, and here I was with my tiny little girl who still had an NG[1] tube,' Gemma told me.

'I think knowing about that world, my previous experience, it helped me accept it much quicker. I was very aware that children die and that my child could, and I accepted that,' she continued.

Now, at last, Gemma felt that her prior experience – of the world of complex medical needs, of paediatric palliative care – gave her a head start. She told me that once they knew what they were dealing with, she was able to accept the input of the palliative team. She'd felt empowered enough to ask to be referred to a children's hospice for support. Her partner was not quite on board.

After a meeting with the palliative team where Zoe's prognosis was discussed together with the options for symptom management,

---

1   Nasogastric tube.

he turned to Gemma and said, 'Well, we probably won't need them, to be honest.' It was then that Gemma realised that they were not on the same page and her partner had not come to terms with his daughter's life-limiting diagnosis.

Gemma's experience as a palliative care nurse now gave her the confidence to push back when she didn't agree with the doctors and nurses. She had already had an insight into this world and what goes on behind the scenes.

But it was just a head start. Zoe is now ten. She still has regular hospital admissions, she's still supported by a children's hospice, and the palliative team are still involved. However, Gemma confessed that she still has many times of feeling frustrated, disempowered and being labelled by the nursing staff as 'that mum'.

Whatever the starting point and level of prior experience, we parents of children with the most complex of medical conditions all eventually seem to reach a point where we become the expert – the expert on our child – and that gives us confidence to be able to push back, to ask questions, to assert ourselves.

Time after time, I was told by other parents – those outside the new world I now found myself in – 'I don't know how you do it. I couldn't be like you.'

It's not as if we were born with some sort of superpower that made us saintly carers overnight; we just had to rise to the challenge and draw from reserves that we didn't know we had.

My answer was always 'I didn't know I could be like me'. I'm just like you – any of you – just an ordinary person thrown into an extraordinary situation, trying to navigate my way through, for the sake of my child.

We all have choices. There are always options. When Daisy was in neonates, a baby was left behind by her parents, put up for adoption because they decided they could not cope with the demands of her disabilities. So there are choices, and you make your choice, then get on with it. For me, the training was the deeply immersive experience of living with a child with medical complexity 24/7. You soon learn to sink or swim.

ANYTHING FOR MY CHILD

And you have to keep swimming because your child relies on you to advocate for them, to make decisions for them, to try to think about what they would want you to do for them.

That's all there is to it: just keep swimming.

CHAPTER 5

Don't Call Me Mum

I'VE SPENT YEARS OF MY LIFE WAITING IN HOSPITALS. Staring at the institutional, magnolia-painted walls. We had only been home for a few weeks after Daisy's two-month stint in the neonatal unit when I found myself waiting in a hospital ward again. Hoping for answers, dreading what they might be.

When we arrived on to the ward at Great Ormond Street Hospital, we were shown to Daisy's room and told a nurse would be along soon. Two hours later, we were still pacing the room, waiting to be seen, waiting for a plan. We were here, after all, because there was a chance that our tiny little baby, only a few weeks out of the neonatal unit, had some sort of cancer.

Daisy needed an MRI scan, but she needed to lie still for it, so that involved a general anaesthetic, and she had to take her turn with all the other sick children who needed the same scan. She had blood tests taken which were sent off to labs all over Europe, and a radioactive isotope was ordered from Germany to conduct a specialist nuclear medicine scan.

An oncologist asked us if it would be OK for a geneticist to come and see Daisy. I shuddered, remembering my experience with genetics only a few weeks before in the neonatal unit. This geneticist was a professor, visiting from Utrecht; he specialised in so-called dysmorphic syndromes and apparently knew a lot about Costello syndrome, the condition that had previously been mentioned in relation to Daisy.

This experience was such a contrast to my previous experience of genetics. He was warm and respectful; he asked my permission to examine Daisy and he explained what he was seeing. He then told me that it was more likely than not that Daisy had Costello syndrome and that as the gene mutation that caused it had now been identified, it would be possible to test her for it.

Costello syndrome is caused by a mutation on an oncogene, a cancer-causing gene. It means that people diagnosed with the syndrome also have an above-average risk of malignancy. But in a typical genetics double whammy, people with the Costello syndrome gene mutation also make higher levels of catecholamines, the hormones that can indicate a tumour, which rendered standard blood tests unreliable. It did mean that if genetic testing confirmed that Daisy had Costello syndrome, she would need to be scanned regularly to rule out the presence of tumours.

The most important thing I remember that genetics professor telling me, however, was to never forget that Daisy was just Daisy. Not a patient, not a diagnosis, just a little girl in a family that loved her.

He gave me some information about Costello syndrome, thanked me for my time and left. I never saw him again, but despite the fact that I had just been given devastating news – the likelihood that my little girl had a life-limiting condition and could potentially not make adulthood – I felt strangely sanguine. A semblance of a plan was beginning to form. We were beginning to know what we were dealing with.

Daisy, in the meantime, was becoming sicker. Her breathing was becoming more laboured with every passing day, and she seemed to be in so much discomfort. Andy was back at work, my older children were at the childminder and school, and my youngest son, still only two years old, spent the days with me in the hospital until Andy was able to collect him to take him home for the evening.

It was a strange life. We were juggling: trying to be parents, trying to understand what was going on with Daisy, trying not to worry our other children who really did seem to take it all in their stride.

They were small enough to think of it as an adventure; there were lots of things to keep them entertained around the hospital, and at home plenty of friends were helping out and distracting them.

Daisy was being closely monitored, her breathing was becoming more and more of an effort, and she lay with her head thrown back to try to get more air into her lungs. Doctors came and went; they checked charts, listened to her chest, made calls to other specialists.

'Daisy needs support to help her breathe,' the ward registrar told me. It was very late at night, and it was clear that Daisy was becoming exhausted with the effort to breathe. The decision was made to transfer her to the intensive care unit, and I quickly found myself hurrying along the empty corridors as my daughter was wheeled ahead in her little cot, nurses and doctors running beside her.

I have a photo of her, taken the next day, pale with plastic bubble wrap to keep her warm, ventilated and still. I was struck by the fact that this was the first time I had seen her lying straight – from very early on, she had thrown her head back and arched her back. She looked peaceful.

There was nothing I could do but sit next to Daisy's cot and watch the monitors flash and beep as nurses busied themselves around her.

Andy was with me, and soon a stream of specialist doctors appeared. We were given diagnosis after diagnosis as each doctor delivered their verdict on what was going on with our daughter. The cardiologists had found she had thickening of the heart muscle; the respiratory doctors were concerned that she had laryngomalacia, a floppy airway, which was contributing to her breathing problems; tests showed that she had severe reflux and was aspirating feed into her lungs; the neurology team thought she probably had a visual impairment...

I had to leave the room. I needed to get some fresh air. It was overwhelming: one after another, these doctors, each representing different specialties, were coming into Daisy's room, dropping bombshells and leaving. I couldn't take it in.

We had thought it was bad a few months ago, when Daisy had arrived in our lives prematurely and sick. Now it was worse: she was ventilated and very poorly, and there were clearly a lot of things going on contributing to that.

Were we ever going to get home again? Were we ever going to just be parents to this child?

Gradually, Daisy got better. She came off the ventilator, and we moved out of intensive care, this time to a neurology ward. She was already on a cocktail of drugs; special formula was now being drip-fed into her stomach via a pump connected to her nasogastric tube. She was slowly being weaned off her pain medications. I could see her growing and developing, responding to familiar voices and, at last, smiling.

One day, as I was leaving the ward to get something to eat, the ward doctor saw I was about to go out and ran after me.

'Mum! Mum!' he called.

I turned around and looked at him, this young, enthusiastic junior doctor, not long qualified, who needed to tell me something about my daughter. I was almost old enough to be his mother. He had Daisy's notes in his hand, the front page of which had our family contact details including my name.

'Don't call me Mum!' I snapped at him.

He was taken aback.

I had become increasingly irritated by this practice of not asking parents or carers their names and just referring to me as Mum – it stings on so many levels. At the time, it was about someone who just assumed that it was OK to call me Mum, but over the years I have found that there is a deeper issue. It's not about being called Mum; it's about not being asked what you want to be called. Did my role as Daisy's parent, advocate, carer, the person willing to take on complex medical training just to get her at home, did that role just boil down to the catch-all of 'Mum'?

Parents of children with complex needs are living this life 24/7; there is no one else more qualified to describe the day-to-day details of their child. Asking what we want to be called is about humanising the interaction and respecting the role that parents play in their child's life. It also ensures that parents feel that they have a seat at the table and are not just an item on the agenda.

I have met many mothers who don't mind being called Mum, and that's fine, but don't assume that's always the case. I remember years later sitting outside a room where a large multi-disciplinary meeting was taking place to discuss Daisy. There were doctors and nurses and therapists around the table, all discussing my daughter's life, and yet the person who lived with her, who knew every minute detail about her routine, her responses, her wants and needs, was on the other side of the door. My role, my experience, reduced to an agenda item which stated – 'Mum to join the meeting at the end'.

Being referred to as Mum immediately created a power-based relationship that did not recognise my role in Daisy's life, in keeping her alive. The hours I spent administering her drugs, managing her therapies, educating myself on the complexities of her rare disease, seeking to understand what she would want me to say if she could speak. I found it beyond frustrating when, again and again, healthcare professionals didn't ask me how I'd like to be addressed, especially during an extended hospital stay.

As one parent told me, 'From a parental perspective, there's so little we can control in hospital, and this is one of those things, so maybe that's why upsets us so much.'

Conversely, another parent wanted me to know that she was OK with being called 'Mum', but as a single parent with only one child, it was for very different reasons:

You know what, I must be the only person who loves it when anyone calls me Mum! Maybe it's because Sammy can't speak so she can't call me that and maybe it's because I don't have other children who can. But I just love being called it. Sometimes my role gets a bit confused and I feel more like an admin person or liaison officer, so anyone calling me Mum reminds me of who I am.

A few years ago, I wrote a piece for the *British Medical Journal*[1] about this subject. It became one of their most shared patient-perspective pieces, and I continue to be contacted by medical professionals who tell me that it was a lightbulb moment – it just had not occurred to them. If we are to foster a culture of collaboration between parents and the professionals caring for their child, then it's about time we stop assuming that referring to 'Mum' or 'Dad' is acceptable. It should be acceptable to ask how a parent wants to be addressed. This changes the dynamic hugely, humanising the conversation, recognising the role played by the person living and caring for the child 24/7.

After all, it's now increasingly the norm that professionals in healthcare settings introduce themselves by name rather than just their role.

The #HelloMyNameIs campaign is an important legacy of the work of the late Dr Kate Granger.[2] Kate was a specialist in geriatric medicine who found herself on the other side of the bed when she was diagnosed with a rare form of cancer. She started the #Hello-MyNameIs hashtag campaign on Twitter after she became fed up with the lack of introductions from medical staff who were caring for her. It felt wrong that such a basic step in communication was missing. Now many hospitals have taken on board the principles of the campaign, and staff are trained to introduce themselves, often wearing easy-to-read name badges bearing their first name.

Kate's premise was about humanising the interaction between the medical professional and patient, focusing on person-centred, compassionate care. It's an important step in moving away from a patriarchal 'doctor knows best' model of healthcare to one of increased patient autonomy. The starting point in Kate's campaign was always about clinicians introducing themselves, but there is a lot more to it than that. She went on to identify four core values that are vital in clinical staff and patient interactions:[3]

---

1   Nimmo, S. (2019) 'Please don't call me mum.' *BMJ* 367. www.bmj.com/content/367/bmj.l5373

2   www.hellomynameis.org.uk

3   www.hellomynameis.org.uk/key-values

- Communication – it starts with a simple introduction: Hello, my name is...

- The little things – they really do matter. Just thinking about how you speak to someone, sit next to them. Don't loom over them, for example.

- Patient at the heart – no decision about me, without me.

- See me – as a person first, not a disease or diagnosis.

Dr Kate Granger started the ball rolling and catalysed a culture change in the NHS. It reminds anyone involved in a patient's care that the simple act of just introducing yourself to a patient is an important step in fostering a culture of collaborative communication.

But there's more that can be done, and it's not just about hashtags and name badges. By taking the time to ask the parent of a child with complex needs – the person tasked with caring for them, advocating for them and keeping them alive – what they would like to be called is a positive first step in fostering a culture of collaboration and humanising communication between parents and professionals.

The comments of a parent I spoke to sum it up:

I would rather be asked what I want to be called, but forgive people who are meeting us briefly. It's not acceptable after eight months living on a ward, though! That's just condescending and lazy. It's also not acceptable in formal meetings where everyone else is being addressed by their names. And in clinic letters, 'Mum said' is used to belittle statements made by parents.

Daisy was three months old when she went into Great Ormond Street Hospital. She came home nearly three months later.

We adjusted to the daily routine of setting up the feed pump, passing tubes into her stomach and administering an ever-increasing range of drugs. The ubiquitous brown envelopes began dropping through the letterbox. Invitations to clinic appointments,

consultant's letters. 'For the parents/guardians of Daisy Nimmo.'
Hospital numbers tripped off my tongue. Weights and measures
were a constant in my life as every pound of weight gained was a
cause for celebration.

Two important letters arrived at our house on the same day.
The first was the confirmation that Daisy did indeed have the gene
mutation that causes Costello syndrome. This life-changing piece
of news was delivered as a postscript in the general letter from the
geneticist who had first examined Daisy in the neonatal unit all
those months ago.

I sat on the stairs with my head in my hands. Now we knew what
was going on. Now we knew that Daisy had a life-limiting condition,
that she might not reach adulthood but would need a lot of input
from a lot of people for the rest of her life, however long or short.
I had visions of my future self, an older woman, tired and worn
out, holding the hand of an adult child, my last child still living at
home, my forever child.

I opened the second letter. Ruth had referred us to our local
children's hospice for support, and this letter confirmed that we
had been accepted and were invited to come and visit. When Ruth
had mentioned a children's hospice, I didn't think about death and
dying. She had framed the referral as a way for us to get some support. We had four children under seven and no close family nearby.
I knew that family life as we had known it was never going to be
the same again. Our children were already beginning to experience
the realities of life as the siblings of a complex child; at least at the
hospice, they could have a bit of a break from that and spend time
with other families who didn't stare or ask awkward questions.

And there was also the very stark reality that Daisy would not
reach adulthood. At that time, we were in the very early days of
genomic medicine. Daisy was one of the first children in the world
to be tested for Costello syndrome and receive a positive diagnosis.

We connected with the Costello syndrome support group and
chatted to other families around the world. Daisy's medical com-
plications already seemed very extreme compared to some of the

other children with the same diagnosis, however. Doctors referred to her as life-limited. We knew deep down that we would need hospice support one day in a very different way – that it would be more than just a place to have a family break together.

When would that endpoint come? Daisy was slowly developing. Her personality was revealing itself. Always happy to be with people, interacting with her siblings, she became the centre of our home. Our children did not see the tubes, the medicine syringes, the therapists who came to visit, the ever-increasing specialist equipment that a physiotherapist would bring to the house. They just saw their sister.

But she cried a lot and seemed to be in a lot of pain. Specialist feed was constantly drip-fed directly into her stomach via a newly formed gastrostomy. Even that supposedly simple procedure had entailed a two-day stay in the intensive care unit. She would spike temperatures or vomit uncontrollably, and I would find myself back in the hospital with her, wondering if this was the beginning of the end. Wondering how much I could dare allow myself to love this child, knowing that one day I would lose her.

It was Andy who snapped me out of it. 'It's like we're in a car, driving along a very long road, bracing ourselves for an inevitable crash,' he said. 'The problem is, we don't know when that crash is going to happen, and while we're bracing ourselves and waiting for it, we're missing incredible scenery that's just outside the window.'

He was right. I was so focused on the future – what was going to happen to Daisy, to our family – that I was missing the here and now: the milestones that she was hitting, our other children growing up, life continuing around us.

So we took off our metaphorical seatbelts and decided to try to enjoy the ride, no matter how long or short it was.

It struck me that our other children only had one shot at childhood, and their needs had to be balanced alongside our worries and concerns. Hospital admissions continued, our worries continued, but in between those, we made huge efforts to just be a family. Our world revolved around Daisy, but we needed the world to revolve around our family so that we could be together to ensure that each of our children got time and had a chance for a childhood.

I think I had always accepted that Daisy would not be with us forever. As I grew to understand how her condition affected her, I couldn't see how she would live into adulthood with so much going on. And so we tried to just live for the moment.

It was never about bucket lists or even making memories. It was about appreciating the little things: sitting together on the sofa watching a film, gathering around the table to share a meal, just sleeping in my own bed with all my children tucked up in theirs under the same roof. The little things – they really are the big things, and enjoying the little things and appreciating the things that I previously had taken for granted became the drivers for everything we did from that time onwards. To be a family, to be together, to be home. It's clichéd, I know, but you don't realise how much you appreciate something, need something, until it's taken away from you.

Sometimes people asked me if I ever wondered what my life would have been like if Daisy had not been born with that sporadic mutation on the HRAS gene – if she had been 'normal'. I just did not allow myself to go there. I simply could not. What was the point? This was Daisy, and this was our life. I couldn't torture myself with thoughts of what she would have been doing if she had not been born with Costello syndrome.

And anyway, there is no such thing as 'normal'. It's a relative concept. As a friend told me very early on, 'Normal is just a setting on a washing machine.'

CHAPTER 6

Life, Limited

What exactly does life-limited mean?
When we were told that Daisy would be life-limited, we knew that she wasn't going to die imminently. It didn't feel as though she had a terminal condition, but it felt as if there was finality in the term. I learned to tell people who asked that she would have a shorter childhood than our other children and that she was teaching us all to make the most of our time together. Later, when my husband was diagnosed with terminal cancer, I realised that she had taught us that life really is finite, and that the only thing we have guaranteed in life is that one day we will die She prepared us for a very hard lesson.

Life-limited can feel like a 'catch-all' label which can mean different things in different cases. The UK children's palliative care charity, Together for Short Lives, has identified four categories of life-limiting and life-threatening conditions.[1]

- Life-threatening conditions for which curative treatment may be feasible but can fail (such as cancer or irreversible organ failure).

- Conditions where premature death is inevitable (e.g. cystic fibrosis and Duchenne multiple dystrophy).

---

1 © Together for Short Lives 'Categories of life-limiting conditions.' www.togetherforshortlives.org.uk/changing-lives/supporting-care-professionals/introduction-childrens-palliative-care/categories-of-life-limiting-conditions. Note: These definitions are due to be updated shortly.

- Progressive conditions without curative treatment options (e.g. Batten disease and Huntington's disease).

- Irreversible but non-progressive conditions causing severe disability, leading to susceptibility to health (this category includes children with severe cerebral palsy or disability following a brain or spinal cord injury).

These are broad categories (and work is currently underway to revisit and update them as so much has evolved in medical science since they were first defined). Looking back, Daisy crossed over more than one of them, especially as her medical needs increased in complexity over the years. We were fortunate to receive a confirmed diagnosis of Daisy's underlying condition very early on; many families might never have that answer. The diagnosis was helpful because it gave us guidance on what to look out for – to screen for tumours, to monitor her heart for any progression of the cardiomyopathy, the thickening of her heart muscle, that had been picked up when she was in intensive care. But the diagnosis did not give us all of the answers.

Daisy's disease was rare – there were only around 200 confirmed cases of Costello syndrome globally when she was diagnosed – and in her time, Daisy did things that were not 'typical' for that syndrome. Issues with feeding normally improve with the syndrome; with Daisy, they worsened. The words of the genetics professor were very relevant: 'She is just Daisy.' She was not a disease or a diagnosis; a syndrome, after all, is just a collection of symptoms and conditions, and she seemed to gather a lot over her lifetime.

I still wonder if there was more going on than Costello syndrome. Over time, multiple biopsies and samples were taken which showed various anomalies, not all of which were present in other children with the same gene mutation. Over the course of her life, Daisy seemed to defy the 'norm' even for this very rare disease.

I was constantly searching for more answers, not because I thought Daisy could be cured, but because the more we knew about why things were happening, the better we could manage those symptoms and care for her. On top of that, I wanted to know more for my other children. Costello syndrome is caused by a sporadic gene mutation. It's not an inherited disease – neither Andy nor I carried a faulty gene that had caused the syndrome. But I often wondered, and still do, whether there was a secondary condition going on that might have contributed to the severity of Daisy's symptoms and so many other things that seemed to not be explained by the Costello syndrome diagnosis. And if there was something else going on, was that caused by a rare inherited condition?

The diagnosis was both a help and a hindrance. It helped us connect to a community of people caring for children with the same syndrome, and it helped us know what to be aware of, but when there were things that were non-typical Costello, no one was able to tell us if this was unique to Daisy or an element of the syndrome that had not been seen before.

Some families never get an answer; they don't know what has caused their child's complexity. They are still complex and still clearly life-limited, however. Their families call them SWANs – syndromes without a name.

I was always fascinated by the science behind Daisy's diagnosis; it helped me cope in many ways – to understand the whys and hows of what was happening. I remember seeing news coverage years previously of the ground-breaking work to unlock the human genome. I knew how important that work was at the time, but little did I realise how much I would be personally impacted by it. Now, more and more families are discovering the genetic cause of their child's condition. I think it gives some comfort, provides answers.

Nikki told me that a few years after Lennon died she received a letter confirming that he'd had a very rare mutation. She discovered that there were a handful of children in the world who had the same mutation, but many did not survive a full-term pregnancy. Ironically, the fact that Lennon was delivered prematurely because of Nikki's pre-eclampsia probably saved his life. She told me that she takes some comfort from that knowledge.

Our lives changed almost as soon as I had a positive pregnancy test result for Daisy. The initial shock of a one-in-four chance of a positive diagnosis of Down's syndrome, followed by invasive testing, a tough pregnancy and premature delivery meant that our lives had been turned upside down from the get-go. Normal was now hospitals, therapies, people in our lives, adjusting to a huge change, let alone getting used to our new addition and becoming a family of six.

I wonder how it would have felt to have had a period of adjustment, time to just be a family before the onslaught of medical care, before life in the goldfish bowl.

Sara's story

When my friend Sara gave birth to her third child, a much-wanted third daughter, there was no indication that anything was amiss. Sara's pregnancy had been uneventful, and baby Livvy arrived on time.

Sara and her husband, Alan, focused on adjusting to their new life with their three little girls. Livvy slept in her cot in her parents' room, and despite some issues with reflux, life was good.

Sara vividly remembers the moment when all of that changed.

'Livvy was about 21 months old. It was the end of February, about lunchtime. Alan was at work, my older girls were at nursery,' she told me.

'Livvy was sitting on the floor of our sitting room and suddenly, as if from nowhere, she just started screaming. It was as if a switch had been flipped. She just screamed and screamed. This was not just a toddler meltdown or the approach of the terrible twos; it was like she was possessed.'

Sara instinctively knew that something was not right. 'I knew it was not just a behaviour thing; it was like her personality had changed overnight – she had gone from being a happy joyful child to one who screamed and could not be consoled.'

Eventually, Livvy was referred to a paediatrician who concluded that the reflux was causing the screaming episodes. Sara felt that there was so much more going on than this, that the doctors were not looking at the big picture. She felt as if she was banging her head against a brick wall.

'Where has her walking gone? Where has her talking gone? Where has the eye contact gone? She used to be so joyful...'[2]

Sara, who now also had a new baby to care for, began to feel more and more isolated and exhausted with the demands of her third child.

To Sara, it seemed as if Livvy had dropped into her own little world. She didn't scream so much now, but she had lost all her words and any ability to make eye contact. She lost all interest in anything or anyone around her.

'I just trusted the doctors to come up with an answer, but it was becoming increasingly clear to me that they didn't have a clue,' Sara told me

Finally, Livvy was referred for a fourteen-day assessment at a child development centre. Sara was relieved. Maybe, at last, they would get some answers; maybe, at last, people would believe her.

Livvy was given a diagnosis of global developmental delay (GDD) – a bit of a catch-all, but at least it gave Sara a focus and she could find ways to help her daughter and maybe rekindle a little of the child that she had lost. The family began to find a semblance of normal.

All that changed one evening. Livvy began to convulse uncontrollably, and she turned blue. That tonic-clonic seizure was to be the first of many.

Now the family found themselves on the hospital roller coaster: 999 calls late at night, emergency medications, fluctuating health, intensive care admissions, difficult conversations, unpredictability...

Eventually, Livvy was diagnosed with Rett syndrome, a rare disease caused by a sporadic gene mutation and mainly affecting

2   Gover, A. (2018) *Living Like Livvy: A Mother's Story about the Girl Who Refused to Be Defined by Rett Syndrome.* CreateSpace Independent Publishing Platform.

girls. Children develop normally until about 18 months of age and then they begin to lose skills. It's a progressive neurodevelopmental disorder, and the course and severity of the condition can vary in each child. Livvy had a severe form of the syndrome.

The confirmed diagnosis of a mutation on the MECP2 pathway for Rett syndrome was a turning point in many ways for Sara. Now she knew exactly what was going on with Livvy. They had gone from a time of normal family life to a period of challenging behaviour and a label of GDD to a confirmed diagnosis of a neurodevelopmental disorder, one that could potentially lead to her daughter's premature death.

'Ironically, I felt for the first time that I was being listened to,' Sara told me. 'I appreciated the honesty of the neurologist who diagnosed Livvy. Other doctors made me feel like a neurotic mother; at last, here was a doctor who completely understood what we had gone through, who saw Livvy as a little girl, a member of a family, not a problem to be solved.'

Sara felt relieved, even when the doctor talked about Livvy's prognosis. Finally, there was a professional who believed her and understood what was going on.

'I remember pouring out my heart to him,' Sara said, 'about how I just knew that something was going on with Livvy, that my instinct was telling me more than they were, but no one was listening, no one was hearing me.'

'I hear you now,' the neurologist told her. And even though he had just given her the devastating diagnosis of her daughter's condition, those four words made all the difference for Sara.

We just want to be heard.

Rosie's story

Rosie has a different story to tell, but her instinct that there was something seriously wrong with her child and no one was listening is exactly the same.

She can pinpoint the moment her life changed forever.

'We'd been to stay with my mum for the weekend. I'd put the boys in their PJs for the drive so that they would be ready for bed,' she recounted. 'Matthias, my oldest, told me his bottom was hurting badly.'

'How bad is the pain?' asked Rosie. 'If your burst eardrum was a ten, then what is this?'

'It's an eight, Mum', Matthias answered. She couldn't see anything, but she thought she felt a strange bulge in his perineum, and with that, Rosie knew that something was not right.

This wasn't a fleeting pain, and her son was not one to exaggerate.

'I took him to A&E,' she told me. 'He was in so much pain.'

What else do you do when your nine-year-old child is screaming in pain, and no painkiller is even touching it?

The paediatric A&E waiting room was crowded, with weekend sports injuries and broken bones. Eventually, they were seen by a triage nurse. She couldn't see anything wrong, and, of course, by then Matthias was no longer screaming in pain. That always seems to happen as soon as you go through the swing doors of A&E – it's almost miraculous.

The nurse said that they could either wait their turn to see a doctor, but Matthias wouldn't be a priority as he seemed to be OK, or they could cross over the hall to see the out-of-hours GP.

'That was my biggest mistake,' says Rosie, 'because he just examined Matthias and then told me to make an appointment with our regular GP on Monday.'

And so Rosie boomeranged back and forth to her GP, and they couldn't feel or see anything. The pain didn't go away; Matthias was uncomfortable sitting down, and night after night, Rosie would put him into a hot bath in an attempt to give him some relief. Finally, after more A&E visits, they got to see a consultant, and Rosie hoped that she would finally have some answers and a plan to help Matthias.

'Aaah, it's a haematoma from a fall,' the consultant told her.

He hadn't even examined Matthias, let alone spoken to him. He sent off forms to request a routine ultrasound scan. 'This was April,' Rosie told me, 'and the ultrasound was booked for June. If I'd gone along with what the consultant told me, if I'd ignored my instinct, my son would have been dead by then.'

Rosie just felt that no one was listening to her. She's a teacher, a mother of four boys, a confident, experienced mother, and yet she felt disempowered and voiceless.

From that first trip to A&E, it took six weeks for Rosie and her husband to eventually discover what was going on with their eldest son.

'I made friends with the doctors' secretaries. I kept calling, kept on it; I was not going to sit tight and wait for that ultrasound. My son was in pain, and I needed to know why,' Rosie told me.

Matthias didn't have a haematoma. Instead, he had a rare, fast-growing prostatic tumour, and time was of the essence. Thank goodness Rosie had trusted her instinct.

Rosie and her husband, Tony, had a short, sharp introduction to the world of medical complexity. Now, hospital and illness had become the norm.

There was talk of proton beam therapy, chemotherapy, surgery. The family dynamic changed: Matthias was a now patient and Rosie was a carer. Rosie and Tony were no longer just Mum and Dad; they had to get up to speed quickly to be the advocates and support their son needed. In the space of six weeks, normal family life as they had known it was turned upside down.

Now, they were putting all their hopes in the team treating their son.

What unites Sara's and Rosie's stories is the frustration with trying to get a diagnosis, to get doctors to listen to their concerns that there was something seriously wrong with their child. That they were not over-anxious mothers. They persevered and their instincts were right. But as Rosie told me, 'We lost so much time trying to persuade the doctors that something was not right with Matthias.' And not just time: as both women found, the time they should have spent caring for their child was spent chasing appointments, persuading doctors to listen to them, trying to get their voices heard.

Until, at last, they got a diagnosis and a plan.

It makes no difference at what point you get plummeted into this world. When you learn that your child has a life-limiting condition, the challenge is the same: navigate the complexity, advocate for your child, get up to speed quickly, work out what needs to be done, spin those plates, hold it together.

All of us – the parents who find ourselves caring for a life-limited, medically complex child – we are just ordinary people, thrown into extraordinary circumstances. We survive by putting one foot in front of the other, day in, day out.

CHAPTER 7

Unwittingly
Becoming a Nurse

A S THE MONTHS WENT BY, Daisy was proving to be resilient and determined to grab life with both hands. At the age of two, she was taking her first tottering steps, she was starting to use Makaton[1] sign language to communicate her needs. She was the centre of our home, and her brothers and sister adored her.

Support services were starting to fall into place, and Daisy went to playgroup for a few mornings a week. It felt as though we were getting into a groove with our new family dynamic.

The hospital was still very much part of our life. Unexplained fevers and vomiting would land her a stay, and even something reasonably straightforward like chickenpox resulted in two weeks as an inpatient on the children's ward. On the whole, though, things were OK.

Daisy was under a few specialist teams now, and not a month went by without some sort of appointment – eye checks, hearing checks, heart checks. Feeding and failure to thrive were still a big issue. Daisy was permanently connected to the pump that drip-fed formula into her stomach, 24/7, but we, and she, just took it in our stride. She still seemed to have episodes of pain and hadn't yet managed a full night's sleep, but we adapted and got on with things.

The Costello syndrome family support group was planning a

---

1   Makaton is a simplified form of sign language using symbols and signs to help people communicate. For more information, see www.makaton.org.

conference in Portland, Oregon, that year and we decided to see if we could get to it. We would have a chance to catch up with other families. Most importantly, it would give us an opportunity to meet with the scientists, clinicians and geneticists who were at the forefront of research into the syndrome. These were ones who knew the most about its manifestations and what potential treatments and therapies might be coming down the line. Concern about Daisy's gastro issues were niggling at the back of my mind. My instinct was telling me that there was something more going on. The literature told me that children with Costello syndrome grew out of their gastro and feeding issues, but Daisy seemed to be getting worse. So far, colonoscopies and tests hadn't yielded anything conclusive beyond reflux and slow motility. We hoped that going to the conference might give us some more concrete answers and possibly even a plan for finding a better way to feed Daisy than a 24-hour milk-pump regimen.

Arriving at the conference in Portland, we were immediately surrounded by families with babies, children, teens and young adults who all had the same characteristics as Daisy.

It felt like a family reunion. Back home, people would stare and ask what was wrong with Daisy, because she looked so different from her siblings and peers. Here, at the conference, she was among children who all looked the same as her. Like cousins, which, in a way, they were – genetic cousins, united by one, very random, very sporadic and very rare gene mutation.

These patient support groups are vital. They give us strength in numbers, amplify our voices. We were lucky that Daisy had a diagnosis. Her disease, while rare, meant we belonged somewhere. Some parents, the SWAN parents without a diagnosis, don't get that.

It was wonderful to meet with all the families face to face at the conference, but it was also clear that Daisy was not following typical Costello syndrome patterns. I remember the other parents being really surprised at how unsettled she was at times, and they shared my concerns that there was something not quite right.

Our meetings with the specialist doctors and geneticists in

UNWITTINGLY BECOMING A NURSE

Portland didn't yield many answers. They gave us advice about screening for abnormalities and also some helpful information on the impact of reduced growth-hormone levels on blood sugars, which might explain Daisy's need to have a constant drip-feed of milk into her stomach. Daisy wasn't a 'typical' child, and it was becoming evident that she was also not a 'typical' Costello child.

Our children noticed it, too. Of course, they loved being at the conference, but they commented on how Daisy was the only one permanently attached to a feed pump.

In September that year, Daisy started at a specialist school for children with visual impairments. It had a brilliant reputation, and many children travelled from far away to be pupils there. We were lucky that it was only a couple of miles away from our home – a serendipitous win in the postcode lottery of disability. Daisy was excited to be starting school, her siblings were excited, we were all excited. I was so happy to reach this milestone, to have all of my children in school at last.

But Daisy's pain episodes and obvious discomfort were increasing. One day she kicked out her foot so hard with the pain that she broke a toe. Exasperated, I took her, once again, to A&E. I had learned early on that it was easier to bypass our local GP and go straight to the hospital for anything like this. Our GP was brilliant and prescribed whatever Daisy needed, but she was so complex and under so many teams that it was just easier to go straight to hospital in the hope that we would get answers or at least be reviewed by a doctor who already knew her. Despite notes kept in the department to keep staff up to date with what was going on with Daisy, I still met with problems, trying to get doctors to listen to my instincts and take me seriously.

'Maybe she's just teething?' was the considered opinion of one very inexperienced junior doctor who reviewed her once.

But my confidence and ability to trust my instincts was growing, together with my knowledge of what was right and what was not right with my little girl. I was learning to be more assertive in my interactions with health professionals, and I could guarantee that the pain my daughter was experiencing was definitely not teething.

One day, Daisy spiked a really high temperature and began to vomit uncontrollably. Bloods were taken, and the decision was made to admit her. My instinct, which hadn't failed me yet, told me that this was going to be a long admission.

In fact, it ended up being nearly 12 months long. After a few weeks in the local hospital, a bed became available at Great Ormond Street Hospital, and she was transferred, thin, pale and sunken-eyed, on to the gastro ward. Tests revealed that Daisy had pan-enteric colitis: she had open, inflamed sores along her entire digestive tract from her oesophagus to her rectum. Her gut was unfeedable, and she was in intestinal failure.

She would now have to receive nutrition intravenously. Total parenteral nutrition (TPN) would now keep her alive, administered into her bloodstream through a central venous line, a permanently tunnelled catheter inserted into a vein with the tip resting just into her heart.

This was new territory altogether. There were so many risks associated with administering TPN and its effects on the liver, and these were compounded by the immunosuppression therapy and steroids that were needed to try to reduce the severity of the inflammation in Daisy's digestive tract.

The biggest risk was sepsis, caused by bacteria entering her bloodstream via the central line. Only three months after starting on TPN, Daisy became septic. It happened so suddenly: one minute she was playing in her cot on the ward of the local hospital where she had been transferred, the next minute she had a temperature of 41 degrees Celsius, was pale and shaking violently.

Her blood pressure was in her boots, dangerously low, and the intensive care team worked hard to stabilise her. I watched them try drug after drug, setting up fluid resuscitation boluses, trying to reverse the awful sepsis that was taking control of her little body. I willed her to pull through, believing that this was the moment when we would lose Daisy. But she rallied, like so many complex children do, and while Andy and I were still reeling from the shock and the suddenness of it all, Daisy recovered to fight another day.

All the time Daisy was in hospital, Andy and I were parenting by rota. He was attempting to manage work, I was trying to be a mum to four very different children. We were trying to advocate for our daughter and make sure that she got every chance possible just to be a little girl again. Most of all, we just wanted her home. We'd created a sort of normality, and we wanted that back, whatever it took.

Eventually, after multiple meetings and consultations, trials of feed, investigations and setbacks, the doctors decided that Daisy would have to come home on TPN. It was to become a permanent part of our life.

Now Andy and I had to pass the hardest test we would ever have to take, harder than any exam we had been previously set: we had to learn how to put up the TPN infusion and to keep our daughter safe at home.

Agreeing that Daisy would come home on TPN was one thing; making it happen would need a huge amount of effort and coordination. Not only would we need to be trained and assessed on putting up Daisy's TPN, but negotiations had to take place with our local commissioning authorities about funding the treatment, and our home had to be assessed as suitable for Daisy to safely return to now that she was TPN dependent.

Orders were placed for the separate fridge to house the huge daily bags of nutrient fluids, the equipment needed to sit up the infusions, the pumps, IV poles, syringes, needles...the boxes and boxes of stuff that would replicate a mini hospital at home.

Andy and I had to undergo a two-week training programme at the hospital, learning how to create a sterile and clean environment, the fundamentals of aseptic non-touch technique in order to prevent infection, the risks that could happen and what to do in an emergency. We learned how to safely put up the infusion and connect it to Daisy's central line every day, how to take her blood for testing and how to change the dressings on her line to keep it clean and safe.

We had already seen and experienced the things that go wrong with caring for a central line and administering TPN; Daisy seemed to have gone through the textbook from the episode where the central line displaced from its position just inside her heart and pumped fluid into her chest cavity making her swell up, to sepsis, to the line breaking.

All these things and more had occurred while Daisy was in hospital on a high-dependency ward. Now we would be at home, managing her care, without the back-up of an emergency alarm. And, of course, when I say *we*, it was mainly me, because Andy was working as a freelance management development consultant, which meant he only got paid for the days he worked, so no compassionate leave or time off. And, of course, we had three other children to think of.

Daisy's central line was now her lifeline; without this, we could not get adequate nutrition into her, and she would eventually starve to death.

The scariest thing I have ever had to do in my life was the first time I connected up Daisy's TPN myself on the hospital ward under the watchful eye of the intestinal failure clinical nurse specialist. My heart was pounding. I knew the risks, and her life was now totally and utterly in my hands.

Andy and I were eventually signed off as competent to administer Daisy's TPN, and after 11 long months, we took her home. We lasted 18 days until she spiked a high temperature, and we rushed her back into hospital with a line infection.

This was now our life. We had thought we had a lot of medical equipment in our home before with the milk pumps for enteral[2] feeding. Now our home was increasingly becoming medicalised, with equipment crammed into every nook and cranny and weekly deliveries of boxes of TPN fluid as well as all of the associated ancillaries needed to manage it.

A nurse accompanied us home to help us with the first evening

---

2   Food administered via the gastrointestinal tract.

of TPN connection, and then that was it: we were alone. No one to call for if something went wrong, it was down to us.

I eventually got into my stride, putting up Daisy's TPN infusions. It's incredible what you get used to. When we started TPN training, I was overwhelmed with everything I had to learn. In the early days, I would refer to my notes to make sure I got everything right. Our other children were left to fend for themselves downstairs as Andy and I worked together to set up the drip each evening. Eventually, it just became second nature. Daisy had returned home on a regimen of sixteen-hour infusions which allowed her a few hours break in the day. Eventually, this crept up, and within a few years she was on 24/7 TPN.

As Daisy's medical care became even more complex, I looked back on those early TPN days fondly. It's all relative. What had felt like such a huge step was eventually something I could do (metaphorically) with my eyes closed. I took on more and more medical skills, and before I knew it, I was able to prepare multiple intravenous antibiotic infusions, manage fluid balances and run through additional fluids, put up intravenous pain medications and a whole assortment of other drugs and treatments. When eventually Daisy had surgery to remove her bowel and to enlarge her bladder, I learned how to manage her ileostomy stoma as well as how to catheterise her Mitrofanoff stoma to empty her bladder.

In all, by the time she died, Daisy had a double-lumen Hickman line into her chest (it was her thirteenth line as so many previous ones had needed replacing because of infections), a gastrostomy stoma which drained bile from her stomach, a jejunostomy stoma into the very top of her small bowel, an ileostomy to drain faecal fluid and a Mitrofanoff stoma which had a permanent catheter into it to drain urine.

These words, these medical terms, tripped off my tongue. I could discuss blood results with doctors and nurses and understood what they all meant and what we needed to do. I could set up complex intravenous infusions and fluids, working out the drug calculations to ensure I was giving Daisy the right dose of medication. I could change stoma bags, gastrostomy and jejunostomy buttons, insert catheters and dress central lines.

I had unwittingly become a nurse. Like so many other parents caring for children with medical complexity, I was prepared to do whatever it took to keep Daisy out of hospital and keep her safe at home.

Being able to do this brought a sense of control and empowerment. It meant that we were not reliant on professionals to manage the practicalities of Daisy's care, but in turn it brought other challenges. I had less time for my children, I had less time just to be Daisy's mummy, I had less time for my relationship with my husband and I had less time for myself.

Sometimes, if Daisy was admitted to hospital, I found myself working alongside the nurses or even filling in because some of them didn't have the training or skills to care for her central line, and there was no other option.

Parents take on these risks and become the unqualified experts on their children. We are tasked with keeping them alive while running on empty ourselves, living in a permanent state of hyper-vigilance. There is no back-up at home; night after night, I would get up to administer a controlled drug to Daisy, knowing that if this was in a hospital setting, there would be another member of staff available to check the dose.

I remember once being woken up in the middle of the night by a registrar who told me that they had accidentally given Daisy the wrong strength of oxycodone and essentially overdosed her. Daisy, who seemed to metabolise drugs very differently, didn't have any side effects other than being very itchy, but I remember thinking as the doctor left me to monitor her overnight (bearing in mind that I was not able to actually go off duty and would need to be awake all day on minimal sleep) that if they can have all the controls on the ward to prevent incorrect drug administration and still manage to get it wrong, what a thin line I was trusted to tread at home, taking on the risk to keep my child safe from harm.

We were sent home and trusted to carry out complex care regimens that would require a trained nurse. Nurses and doctors had emergency alarms to press and people to call if things went wrong. They could go home and have an undisturbed night's sleep. I would fall into bed just hoping that I'd got everything right, that I hadn't accidentally administered an incorrect dose of a powerful drug or unwittingly made a fatal error with a piece of equipment.

As my friend Saira told me:

> The best professionals are always the ones who have bothered to actually come to your home and see the set-up. It's absolutely terrifying coming home after a long admission with your child having very different care needs. Unfortunately, we have no choice but to just get on with it, but I do believe it all has a long-term effect on parents.

Katie, a TPN mum friend, ended up having a seizure from the utter exhaustion of the back-to-back intravenous infusions she had to manage just to be able to get her son home and out of hospital:

> Looking back, I would never ever do it again... I say that, but if it meant living in hospital or being at home with my kids together, I guess I'd probably give in and do it again. One thing I do say is that I was never able to be a mum, to either of the kids. Rory could be screaming, and I couldn't cuddle him because I was mid-IVs pretty much all the time. Looking back, it devastates me, because had I lost him as he was so sick, I had no precious time – it was spent doing IV after IV. At the time, I felt it was the right thing just so we could all be together when he was well enough to be at home, but now it just makes me angry. I feel let down actually; it was a ridiculous responsibility. I coped, but I don't know how I did it. Two hours' sleep at night where no IVs were running. My health now, I think, has suffered from the lack of sleep I lived on.

No nurse worth their registration would be prepared to work the hours and undertake the procedures that parents caring for medically complex children are expected to take on without back-up and support. We're invisible. And if our child is not blocking an inpatient bed, then we are very much out of sight and out of mind.

CHAPTER 8

Alone in the Crowd

A DVANCES IN MEDICAL SCIENCE mean that medically complex children are surviving longer. They are leaving hospital
and going home, when previously they would have died. But they
are going home on increasingly complex care and therapy regimens
in order to stay alive, and the burden of care inevitably falls on their
parents to manage this.

It creeps up on us, and before we know it, we become experts
in a range of skills that many medical professionals have little day-
to-day experience of. Daisy's TPN consultant was great at working
out her nutritional requirements alongside her specialist intestinal
failure multi-disciplinary team. But I doubt that she could set up
the pump and drip to administer the fluids and troubleshoot the
problems that I dealt with day in, day out...

It just seems to happen: you take on the biggest challenge
of your life, turn your home into a hospital, put parenting on
the back burner and become the expert on your child's care. Just
to have them at home again. We all have choices. I've been on
wards where children are waiting for specialist foster parents to
come and pick them up because, for whatever reason, their birth
parents are unable to manage the burden of their care. I know
many parents who have adopted children with complex medical
needs. It is a choice, and it's a life-changing choice, to take on a
complex care regimen.

Annette's story

I met Annette at the children's hospice. She came along to the playgroups and family days with her daughter, Sophie. By the time I knew Annette, Sophie, who was a couple of years younger than Daisy, had a tracheostomy which was permanently connected to a ventilator.

Sophie was seemingly fine at birth; she developed normally for the first few months and gave her parents no cause for concern. A chest infection that didn't seem to be getting better was dismissed as 'just a virus' by the GP, and Annette felt she was being an over-anxious first-time mother.

However, 'the virus' became worse. Eventually, when a GP heard Sophie's stridor – the high-pitched wheezing sound caused by a disrupted airflow into her lungs – he immediately sent her for assessment at the local hospital A&E. That was the point at which everything changed.

'She's a bit floppy.' The casual comment of one doctor examining Sophie led her father, Neil, to start Googling the term 'floppy baby'. Sophie was transferred to a specialist paediatric neurology centre.

Test after test ensued, none yielding any positive answers as to why Sophie was becoming more and more floppy and struggling to breathe. After a few long months, she was discharged home – a very different baby now. She needed oxygen and regular suction, had high blood pressure and reflux, and was fed via an NG tube. Annette and Neil were reassured by the fact that the specialist hospitals had not found anything of consequence in all the testing and hoped that Sophie would just get better.

But those hopes were dashed when, during a hospital stay, Sophie suddenly went into respiratory arrest. She was resuscitated and placed on to a ventilator to help her with her breathing. Weeks went by and Sophie was still on the ventilator, unable to maintain her airway, unable to breathe for herself.

Sophie was fully conscious and was clearly uncomfortable with the temporary endotracheal tube which was inserted via her nose into her airway so that she could breathe. It was decided that she should have a tracheostomy; while she was asleep under general anaesthetic, the doctors would also take a full-thickness biopsy of her muscles to see if that would shed any light on what was happening.

'The results of the muscle biopsy came back, and it was bad,' Annette told me, 'so bad that the doctor told us that if they had known the results beforehand, they would never have performed the tracheostomy and would have recommended extubating Sophie and letting her die.'

'That doctor's comment will forever haunt me,' Annette told me. 'It was all about timing, and a slightly different version of events would have meant Sophie wouldn't be here and we wouldn't be having this conversation.'

The doctors don't have all the answers, but I was left to wonder how Annette felt about how a simple timing of a surgery, before the muscle biopsy, had resulted in this. Obviously, she would not change Sophie for the world – she is a much-loved daughter who brings her parents such joy – but Annette's life could have been very different. She would have been a grieving, bereaved mother, but maybe she would have had other children, she could have continued her career, she would not have to share her home with a team of carers. She would not have to go through all that still knowing that her daughter is likely to have a shortened life.

On speaking to other professionals and families, it's clear that it's not unusual for some medical decisions to be seen as having more ethical significance than others. Tracheostomy, and the decision on whether or not to perform the surgery, often seems to be a particularly important decision. But not all agree. I spoke about this, in relation to Sophie's case, with an ethicist, and he expressed concern at the idea that it was not possible to move to palliative care after having performed a tracheostomy. He felt that this was a mistaken approach. What mattered ethically for Sophie at the time was the nature of her underlying illness, her parents' priorities for her care and, fundamentally, her 'best interests'.[1] That isn't changed by the position of her breathing tube (in her neck rather than her mouth), and she could have been transitioned to a palliative care pathway even after the tracheostomy.

The decision on whether a permanent tracheostomy and breathing support was the right course of action was now no longer relevant. Sophie had a permanent breathing tube in place, and the doctors began to discuss plans for her to go home on a ventilator. Now Neil and Annette's life would revolve around the care of Sophie's airway at home. Now they would be responsible for keeping her alive.

The couple were told it could potentially take up to ten months to put in place the package of care and support they would need to be discharged, but they were also acutely aware that Sophie's prognosis was not good, that she was life-limited and unlikely to reach adulthood.

Once again, it fell to a personal recommendation, a 'someone who knows someone' scenario, to change things for the family. So many friendships are formed from adversity, especially when you are a parent of a child with complex needs and spend more time in a hospital parents' room than in your own home. Annette was in the parents' room of the intensive care unit one day chatting to one of the other mums on the ward. She poured out her frustrations about the time it was going to take to get Sophie home and how she hated the thought of what could potentially be their last months together with their daughter being spent on a hospital ward.

'Have they mentioned the children's hospice?' the other mother asked Annette. 'There's one really close to your home, and surely Sophie could be transferred there while you wait for the local services to approve all the funding.'

'It turned out my friend knew many of the team at the hospice,' Annette told me.

So calls were made, and within days Sophie was transferred. Life

---

1   I discuss this in greater detail in Chapter 16.

improved immeasurably. Annette and Neil were able to do things they had only been able to dream about while they were in hospital. They took Sophie swimming in the hydrotherapy pool, chilled out as a family on the sofa, basked in the sunshine in the garden.

The hospice nursing team began to train up the supporting home care team that would be needed for Sophie to return home safely, and after two months, Annette and Neil were able to bring their little girl back home. Annette, like me, did not return to work after her maternity period ended.

Now there were carers in the house, staying overnight in Sophie's room for six nights a week. Their home was filled with equipment, and Annette became the expert on ventilator settings, on how to change Sophie's tracheostomy and gastrostomy tubes. Doing everything to keep Sophie at home and out of hospital has involved recreating some elements of hospital life at home.

'I remember coming home and feeling totally and utterly overwhelmed,' she told me. 'We had gone from a quiet two-bed Victorian semi to a busy house full of equipment and people. I used to say the house felt like a bus station with people constantly leaving and arriving. And the equipment meant we really did have a mini intensive care unit in our dining room. It was quite surreal – like we were living in some kind of parallel universe. We were not in contact with any other families at the time, so we didn't have anyone to talk to who was in a similar situation. We felt isolated, yet we were surrounded by people. It was (and still is) a lonely place to be.' Annette hit the nail on the head there.

Adjusting to carers was a huge challenge. Annette describes how their home was no longer their home – it was a 'workplace'. She and Neil had to constantly monitor what they said and did in front of the team caring for Sophie. This was not helped by the fact that the layout of the house meant that to get to the kitchen or bathroom, they would have to pass through the dining room, which was now Sophie's bedroom. Imagine how that feels. Every midnight snack, late-night wandering, argument...constantly under scrutiny. Knowing that when you shut the front door, you could not simply relax.

When Daisy came home on TPN, we were not offered a care package. And being naive at the time we thought we could just get on with things. We were so grateful to be going home. It didn't occur to us that we would need help in managing Daisy's care, and it seemed that it didn't occur to anyone to offer it.

It was years before we were offered any help. Daisy's care had become increasingly complex, and an assessment was made to put in place a package of nursing support to help us. It's such a postcode lottery. We had to get to breaking point to be able to have funded support, whereas some families leave hospital with it all in place ready for them.

Accepting this intrusion into our lives just to be able to get some sleep and rest is the price we pay to be at home and out of hospital, and eventually you just learn to live with it. For Annette, the days and weeks passed, and things got easier and they were able to form some sort of a routine. After six months at home, she managed to leave the house with Sophie and drive her to places with a carer next to her in the back of the car. At last, she felt part of the world again and was able to give Sophie an insight into life outside walls.

Annette told me that she will always be immensely grateful to the carers and nurses who supported the family. 'They gave us sleep, a break, and taught me how to learn to enjoy spending time with my little girl and forget the machines. I know this comes easy to most parents, but, for me, it was blurred by hospital stays, equipment and anxiety. I worried that every day with her might be my last.'

Like me, Annette learned to enjoy the journey and unbuckle her seatbelt.

Sophie is now a teenager. She is defying her statistical odds, and she is also demonstrating considerable intellectual insight. Although she's unable to move independently and is still dependent on her ventilator, technology is supporting her in other ways. She is able to use a special switch-based communication system, which means she can tell people around her how she feels and what she needs. When I was interviewing Annette for this book, she showed me copies of messages that Sophie sends her – coherent, clear, insightful and opinionated communication, from a teenage daughter to her mum.

Nobody knew what the future would be like for Sophie when she was discharged home. It comes back to that academic guesswork comment, the fact that when dealing with this level of complexity, it's impossible to give a prognosis, make a definitive decision on life expectancy. Perhaps we're just wrong to be focusing on this. How long is my life-limited child going to be here? How long have we got together? The more we know about genomic medicine, the more we understand how patients can respond very differently to a treatment or therapy despite having the same diagnosis.

The more we know, the less we know as well, because what works for one person or what is statistically a prognosis for one is not for the other. And as Stephen Jay Gould wrote in his essay 'The median isn't the message',[2] there is so much more at play than statistical odds to determine survivability.

I vividly remember the first night we had a nurse come to the house to care for Daisy. This had followed years of broken sleep, and I was on my knees. Andy sometimes had to travel with his job. He was also now freelance after having accepted a voluntary redundancy package, so while it gave us flexibility, it also meant no pay on the days he didn't work.

Our other children were growing up, and they had their own issues. We had recently had confirmation that our elder son, Theo, was autistic. In later years, we were to discover that his younger brother, Jules, had a form of autism called pathological demand avoidance, and to complete the set, it was years later, at 21, that my elder daughter, Xanthe, received a confirmed diagnosis of ADHD.[3]

By this point, Daisy was on her TPN pump for around 18 hours a day. While she was on the pump, she could only be cared for by either Andy or me or a qualified nurse, trained in the care of central venous lines. In the time she was not on the pump, she went to

2   Gould, S.J. (2013) 'The median isn't the message.' *Virtual Mentor 15*, 1, 77–81. doi:10.1001/virtualmentor.2013.15.1.mnar1-1301
3   Attention deficit hyperactivity disorder.

school, and I had a break of sorts. As much of a break that you can have when you're catching up with all the washing and life admin that's involved with the care of a child with complex needs, let alone neurodiverse children.

Daisy also now had an ileostomy stoma. The gut rest from the TPN had helped to some extent, but the inflammation was still there, and her large bowel had been removed to try to manage the haemorrhaging and a stoma formed. The surgeon told me that when he operated on Daisy, her colon was falling apart in his hands. Biopsies showed that the ganglions, the nerves that make the gut work, were ectopic – it was like having a car with a perfectly working engine that had just been shoved on to the roof.

I fought and fought for help and support. I was washing bedding constantly, weekends were a trial to be endured, and without the hospice and the respite they were occasionally able to offer, I don't know how I would have coped. I remember saying to our community nurses that surely to be able to sleep was a basic human right. That prisoners seemed to have more rights than parents caring for children with complex needs, alone and out of sight. Children on TPN need to have a trained nurse with them while their infusion is running; they cannot be left with a carer if the trained parent is not around. Ironically, if Daisy had a tracheostomy and was not on TPN, then we would have been entitled to a full package of care. It seemed that the rules for how TPN-dependent children should be cared for in the community had not caught up with reality. Providing nurses to care for Daisy was about four times more expensive than providing carers for a child on a ventilator, and I was made very aware by the local budget holders about how expensive my daughter's package of care was.

I didn't want to have to hand over Daisy's care to anyone else (or at least anyone other than our trusted hospice nurses), but I also needed a break...I needed sleep. Daisy had never been a good sleeper, but the broken nights were getting worse. Now it wasn't just about getting her to sleep and trying to grab what sleep I could. She would sometimes need a course of intravenous antibiotics or an additional infusion, and I'd have to set an alarm to set this up, sleepy-eyed and myopic, praying that I'd got it right.

Eventually, we got word that funding had been agreed to provide a nursing care package for two nights a week. We greeted the news with a mixture of elation and trepidation.

The doorbell rang that first evening. All I knew was that a nurse called Anna had been allocated to Daisy's package of care, and she would be coming to our home for a couple of nights a week, staying for an eight-hour shift. I'm so grateful that our first experience of home nursing was with Anna. She was a very experienced Australian nurse, and she was just brilliant at putting me at ease. I immediately knew that we were in safe hands. Even more importantly, Daisy adored her. Gradually, more nurses were added to Daisy's care package, and we learned to live our lives with someone else in the house. Daisy's room was next to our bedroom, and I had to just let go and get used to the fact that while I was asleep, someone was awake in the room next door with my daughter.

It was tough, our lives on display like never before, people coming and going, but there was no choice. We were lucky to even have a homecare package; I knew many families who were struggling. Eventually, when Daisy's condition deteriorated to the point that her TPN had to run 24 hours a day, she would be accompanied to school by a nurse. I had other children, and they needed me. In many ways, that was fortunate because I had to accept nurses into our lives and to care for Daisy so that I could also be there for my other kids.

Andy and I often felt as if we were like ships that passed in the night, juggling childcare, work, life admin. We had no time for each other anymore: life revolved around caring. Daisy's health was so unpredictable, and there were numerous times when plans were changed at the last minute. The children got used to coming home from school to find that Daisy was back in hospital, but we worked hard to make sure that at least one of us (normally Andy) held the fort in some way back at home. It was parenting by rota at times. At least when the night nurse arrived, we could have a few minutes of normality. We were not allowed to leave the house when nurses were on duty, though, so date nights were pretty few and far between. We were driven by our determination to enjoy the journey, however, always making most of the little things, taking nothing for granted.

But respite, nursing and carer packages – none of this was automatic. Everything had to be fought for, budgets balanced; our lives with Daisy were broken down by the hour and every hour was costed out. Members of the community nursing team would come to our house armed with questionnaires, reducing the care we were giving at home to a series of categories all with points attached. To be eligible for a continuing care package of nursing support, we had to hit a certain number of points. I was so frustrated. Why was the process so automated? I knew it was about public money, but why, for example, did a child who needed oxygen via non-invasive ventilation qualify for more hours of care than Daisy who needed TPN 24/7. And why was it such a postcode lottery? I discovered that a child living five miles away from us was eligible for more funded nursing hours, despite needing less care, just because he lived in a different commissioning area.

It seemed as if the assessment forms and systems had not caught up with the advances in medical technology. Being at home full-time on 24/7 TPN was not a very common occurrence, so Daisy's nutritional needs were categorised as severe feeding difficulties for the purpose of the form. But she had complete intestinal failure: this was something so much bigger than *feeding difficulties*.

It felt at times that we were the only ones who knew the big picture – the impact of these complex regimens on our day-to-day lives. The specialist doctors who make the decisions to add in more medications, increase our workload, don't know what life is like for us at home. They don't even know what our homes are like; they assume the community-based services sort all of that side out. The joined-up communication between all of the services is simply left to the parents at the centre to piece together. To know who does what, to tell people what should be happening.

Thank goodness Ruth had referred us for hospice care at the

beginning of our journey with Daisy, because I just don't know how we would have coped otherwise.

Gradually, more and more funded support began to fall into place, but it took years, and looking back at pictures of Andy and me during that time, I can see the toll it took. Carers are exhausted. We fight all the time, we fight for basic rights – the right to sleep, the right for our child to have an education, the right for our other children to have a childhood, the right to step back from always being on duty and just to be our child's parent.

CHAPTER 9

A Seat at the Table

W E'RE TRAINED TO RESUSCITATE OUR CHILD. We are told the risks of getting things wrong, and we are entrusted with keeping our child alive. We have to switch off our parenting instinct and become a nurse.

> I was terrified! Terrified of making a mistake that could cost Sophie her life and that it would be my fault. It was a HUGE responsibility to take on. I remember sobbing quietly on a number of occasions. (Annette, Sophie's mum)

Living with this knowledge, it's difficult to let go. It's difficult to allow someone else to take over your child's care. At home, it is a little easier. The nurses and carers are normally the same, so you start to build up a team, and there is some control about who is going to be caring for your child. Plenty of parents will share stories of carers who were supposed to be on a waking night shift – in other words, awake while your child sleeps – who fell asleep, discovered when a parent popped their head around the door because of the snoring.

I remember one new nurse starting on Daisy's care package, and instantly I did not feel right about her. I would normally take over care so that the nurse could watch me if they were new to our team; then, a few shifts later, I would watch them as they set up the intravenous infusions and changed the TPN bag. But this nurse seemed to lack confidence and really did not know what she was doing. I stayed awake all that night because I could not trust her to keep Daisy safe.

Leaving your child in the care of nurses in respite or on a hospital ward – that's a completely different level altogether. Our nurses were not allowed to care for Daisy when she was in hospital; as far as the commissioning team were concerned, she was being cared for by nurses on the ward, so they did not pay for nursing care during the times when Daisy was an inpatient.

Except we all know that for children with complex medical needs, who need a very complicated care regimen and need to be monitored constantly, being on a hospital ward, especially in a general hospital, is not the safest environment unless a parent stays.

This is where things can get really complicated. At home, we're used to running things with our team, on our timetable; once back on a ward, we have to step back and be 'mum' again. I was fortunate that we were in and out of hospital so much that the staff knew me and knew Daisy; protocols were in place, and I was allowed to manage a lot of Daisy's care, putting up her TPN and infusions. It was a battle hard won, and a bit of a pyrrhic victory really, because it meant that when Daisy was in hospital, I really did not get a break. Forget about the fact that my daughter being in hospital meant that she was ill or undergoing some procedure, test or surgery; I was having to manage her care while speaking to doctors, therapists and nurses, fielding calls from home and trying to keep Daisy entertained and distracted.

I remember one time when Daisy was an inpatient, I was exhausted and had managed to get a bed for the night off the ward, in the parents' accommodation block. My phone rang at 7.30 the next morning.

'Hi – what's wrong?' I asked, immediately assuming the worst.

'Hi, Steph. Just checking – can you make sure you get to the ward for eight, please? A couple of our nurses have called in sick, and we don't have enough cover to care for Daisy...'

No wonder parents are grumpy, distracted, annoying or even rude. I would try to explain to student nurses and junior doctors that we're not like the average parent you see rocking up at A&E

who may have only had a few nights of missed sleep with a child who has only just become unwell.

No, we are living 24/7 in a state of permanent hypervigilance: we're exhausted, our antennae are up constantly, we are juggling trying to be our child's advocate with also trying to be a good parent. We may have other children we are worried about, and they may have their own issues. We will have relationship problems (show me any relationship that doesn't run into problems when one parent is permanently based at hospital and the other is trying to keep things running at home). We may have a pounding headache because we haven't had a caffeinated drink (the lifeblood of the special needs parent) or anything other than vending machine snacks all day because we can't leave our child's side. We exist on microwave meals and minimal daylight, and the soundtrack to our lives is often the theme tune to *Fireman Sam* or *PAW Patrol*.

We are existing.

And we can't always be happy, smiley people. After all, at least you get to go home and sleep.

Hospital sleep for parents of medically complex children, if we're lucky, is in a bed (sometimes it's just a chair) on a plastic-coated mattress next to our child. Trying to sleep with the light on while doors bang outside and nurses talk in daytime voices or come up to check on your child's observations or set up an IV becomes a skill in itself.

Sometimes you hit the jackpot, and you get to stay in parent accommodation or even go home for a night or two, but you can't sleep because the phone could go at any moment calling you back to the ward: 'Hi, Steph, sorry to bother you, but Daisy's not good at all. It looks like we'll have to transfer her to intensive care...'

'I'm supposed to be one of them,' Gemma, the former children's nurse, told me, 'but they just see me as that "difficult" parent – not everyone, but some of the nurses who don't like it when I question why meds haven't been given or why something hasn't happened.'

'We're trained to protect our child's central line,' another mum whose child was on TPN told me. 'We have to be the only ones

ANYTHING FOR MY CHILD

accessing it to set up TPN when our child is in hospital, but what if we're in a hospital that doesn't know us because there are no beds at the local, and their policies don't allow parents to manage care. No wonder we get labelled as difficult.'

I remember one particularly low point (of many) when Daisy was well enough to be transferred from Great Ormond Street Hospital post-surgery back to our local hospital. Andy was at home and was in agony with kidney stones. He was practically passing out with the pain but had to grit his teeth as he had the three older children at home with him. The ambulance to transport Daisy back to our local hospital, where I would at least be a bit closer to home and have a chance of sorting out a rota of friends to help out, was delayed, by hours.

I was sitting with Daisy, our bags packed, the latest boxes of drugs dispensed, with no idea when she would be transferred. It was getting later and later, and I was exhausted. My poor child, who had not long ago had major surgery, was exhausted and cross. I was worried about what was going on at home. I was hungry, and to cap it all, my period had arrived. I remember sitting on the cold stone stairs outside the ward, sobbing and sobbing. I felt so alone and helpless. I wanted someone to just sort it out and make it better, but no one was doing it. I watched the nurses gossiping at their desk, totally unaware of the mental agony I was going through. It felt unbearably cruel and sad.

The point of that story is to show that there is always something going on under the surface that triggers behaviour. I could have kicked off, shouted at the staff to sort things out. That day, I chose to sob quietly in the corner because it really was so overwhelming. But for parents who are living this life 24/7 – trying to keep our child safe and well, to keep them alive, trying to navigate a complex system that feels so alien, often on very little sleep and while we're trying to spin multiple plates in the rest of our lives – our experiences will shape our response.

Parents will all respond differently. Some will get angry, some will complain, some will grin and bear it until they suddenly explode. But I can guarantee that in every case there will have been an early tipping point, an incident, a throwaway comment, an action or inaction that will ultimately trigger how a parent responds to the teams treating their child.

We have to oscillate: one moment we are the one in charge of our child's care at home, knowing the subtleties of their symptoms and how quickly things can change; then, in another moment, we are expected to trust other people to care for our child when we are not there, trust that they will be able to keep them safe.

No wonder we are anxious about entrusting someone else to get it right. Are they using the correct aseptic non-touch technique when connecting her TPN? Am I confident that they know how to change my son's tracheostomy tube? Will they recognise her pain signals and respond appropriately?

We are 'medical parents'. We know the intricacies of our child's life; we know their medical history, their story. But even when a doctor or a nurse defers to us for information on our child, the system as a whole doesn't always value the input that we bring to the table.

With complexity comes meetings. Lots and lots of meetings. Everything seems to involve a meeting and one of the most common is the multi-disciplinary team (MDT) meeting. With so many people involved in Daisy's care, these became a common occurrence.

MDTs would take ages to set up, trying to pull together all those specialists, trying to establish whether doctors or nurses from the local hospital would come along to participate, trying to get a joined-up viewpoint. Eventually, there would be enough consultants available for a meeting to be held.

And I would sit outside the room, anxiously wondering what was being discussed, waiting to be summoned inside.

My role was an item on the agenda. I was not given a seat at the table.

The format of the meeting is to get everyone around the table to discuss the child's care and agree on a way forward. The first part of that would be to make sure that all of the professionals aired their concerns or disagreements with colleagues in private. Fine. The plan was then for collaborative planning with parents. But the reality is very different from the theory. Often the consultants in the meeting room would forget that I was outside, or maybe they were just pressed for time. They would reach the part of the agenda that involved inviting the parents in. This was at the end of the meeting, and at that point I was told what had been decided and asked my view. The room was half empty by then as they all needed to be somewhere else.

I was lucky: we got to have a few MDT meetings. Consultants actually met together to discuss Daisy's care, and I occasionally got to participate. Talking to other parents, this is not a common occurrence, although health professionals believe it is. How can decisions be made about the care and management of a child with medical complexity without giving time to the person living with that child 24/7, the person living with the impact of decisions on care regimens, the impact on the wider family life, the emotional impact on the child – the person tasked with keeping the child alive?

MDTs, when they did take place, were daunting. I am educated, confident, articulate, an experienced parent, and even I felt anxious walking into a room full of professionals who were responsible for my child. If I felt like that, how would someone who maybe doesn't have English as a first language or is not used to holding their own in a meeting feel? I can't even remember being offered the chance to bring a friend or advocate, or discuss what I wanted to achieve from the meeting. I wasn't given any guidance on what to expect and how to ensure that my view and that of my daughter were heard.

A nurse friend told me recently that some professionals also find these meetings daunting, and it can be why they come across as aloof. But some professionals consistently do not show up, and it's often the usual suspects around the table.

Doctors tell me things have changed, but I'm not so sure. When I ask parents, they have different views. MDTs either happen without them or don't happen at all, or when they do, they feel a bit like lip service. I felt I had to push for the meeting, to try to get a coordinated care plan; it was not something that happened automatically.

Many of the parents I have spoken to have never experienced an MDT or maybe only experienced one or two. Those who have had regular MDTs dread them; it feels like 'them and us' with no chance to influence the agenda and discuss possible outcomes. And sometimes the people who need to be there – community paediatricians, doctors from the local hospital, social workers, teachers –are not invited or can't attend, which means that there's not a full view of the impact of what is being discussed. After all, if the outcome of a meeting is to agree that the child should have a catheter and fluid corrections, how will that work if they are going to school?

'I've always felt talked at, rather than listened to,' one parent told me. 'They are so nerve-wracking beforehand, too, and you go in with a list of questions, which a lot of the time you don't get to work through during the meeting.'

I bang on about this a lot when I speak to medical professionals. We deserve a seat at the table. We are not doctors or nurses (in most cases) – it's important that parents remember that, too – but we are the experts in how to care for our child, and we know what they are like every single hour of the day. We never ever get to switch off – even if they are in respite, we are waiting for the phone call to say they've spiked a temperature or there's a problem with a piece of equipment. We know the impact on the family unit of decisions that are made about their care and the impact on our lives. We are the ones with the big-picture view of who does what in our child's life; it falls on us to coordinate that, across hospitals, across disciplines, school, community.

Co-production is the buzzword at the moment in healthcare, but is it really happening? Are the outcomes of meetings and conversations achievable? Do they recognise the needs and wishes of the family and child? Are their voices being heard?

All too often parents don't feel that they are participants in the conversations about their lives, because that's what these conversations are, after all – about lives, about a family, no matter how big or

ANYTHING FOR MY CHILD

small. So when we are not involved as equal partners about decisions about our children, when our children are not consulted about their wishes (when they are able), when we are labelled as 'difficult' or obstructive, it's important to remember that we don't get to go home and switch off. We don't have a choice. Well, we could walk away, but not many do. We live in a state of hypervigilance, navigating a complicated system, trying to be an advocate as well as a parent. There's no training for what we do, no rule book. We learn skills we never thought we would learn; we learn to interpret medical data that's relevant for our child. Our homes become hospital rooms, and we open up our lives to strangers. We spin plates every single day. We smile, we try to be nice, despite the lack of sleep or the feeling that no one is really listening.

And it could be you. We are all human beings – just an accident, a gene mutation, a cancer diagnosis away from life on the other side, after all.

CHAPTER 10

One Shot at Childhood

'I 'LL NEVER FORGET THE COMMENT you used to make,' Daisy's social worker told me at her funeral. 'Our children have only one shot at childhood, too; it's not just about Daisy.'

This was something I was incredibly aware of. I think back to my reaction when I was first told, in the earliest stages of my pregnancy with Daisy, that I had a one-in-four chance of having a child with Down's syndrome. My initial thoughts had turned to how this would impact my other children, and what it would mean for them to grow up with a disabled sibling.

Our three children were seven, five and two when Daisy arrived in their lives. Not only were Andy's and my lives changed forever, but so were those of our children. Things would never be the same for them. Jules, the youngest, has no memory of life before Daisy, and for the other two, it's pretty hazy. Life from before Daisy was even born, while I was an inpatient hoping not to give birth prematurely, revolved around hospitals.

I have learned that children are resilient and take it in their stride, but also I know, as their mum, that this was not the childhood I wanted for them. Daisy was the centre of attention; she took so much of our time and our emotional energy and the impact and ripples of that ran deep and wide.

Did I want my five-year-old daughter to take pride in being able to tube-feed her little sister? Did I want my two-year-old son to spend his days in a hospital playroom instead of at a playgroup?

Did I want my seven-year-old son to spend his evenings after school at friends' houses rather than in the comfort of his own home?

I know that some of the things they experienced have given them the resilience and empathy that they display today. But if I could have protected them from that, if we could have taken a more straightforward path in life, I would have chosen it. At the same time, however, whenever I reflect back on everything that has happened I would still choose that part of my life that had Daisy in it.

Hindsight is a wonderful thing, and we really don't have an idea what life will throw our way.

Chloe's story

Chloe is a 23-year-old young woman. She graduated with a degree in sociology and is currently working as a teaching assistant in a school for children with special needs.

I remember the first time I saw Chloe. She was just about to turn seven; her sister, Isobel, had been born on New Year's Day. The doctors had transferred Isobel to the neonatal unit as they were concerned about her jaundice.

It turned out that Isobel had a lot going on – a rare genetic syndrome and a liver condition called biliary atresia. A procedure to try to save Isobel's liver failed, and eventually she underwent a liver transplant, receiving the organs from a donor.

'I remember the first time I met Isobel,' Chloe told me. 'I remember holding her, but I don't remember much about those early days. What I remember is the year she spent post-transplant, in intensive care, and the years after.'

Chloe's mum stayed close to Isobel in family accommodation near the hospital, and Chloe and her dad would join her on the weekend.

'I knew every corridor in that hospital,' she told me. 'My dad and I just walked around. It just became part of my life – go to the hospital on Friday, see Mum and Isobel, come home on Sunday with Dad, go to school. I just kind of accepted it – the boredom, the other kids you'd meet in the hospital playrooms, it was just how my life was'.

Chloe reflected, 'I don't think I fully grasped how sick my sister was until my late teens. I knew my baby sister was very ill, I knew she was very yellow. I knew my mum lived at the hospital and I only saw her at the weekends, and that Isobel spent a lot of time in intensive care, but I don't think I realised how close she was to dying.'

Chloe told me that she looks back now and, at the time, she didn't realise how different her life was – seeing her sister, post-transplant, in intensive care, open wounds to allow the new liver space to adjust. 'I mean, I looked at my sister and could see her open abdomen,' Chloe recalled. 'The surgeon let me hold her old, diseased liver that he'd just removed, in a plastic bag in my hands – that's just not a normal childhood experience, is it?'

Isobel was referred to the same hospice as Daisy. By the time she left hospital, she had a tracheostomy and her wheelchair was laden with emergency equipment. The hospice referral meant that not only could Isobel have time to just be a little girl, safe in the care of nurses who knew how to manage her needs, but Chloe had some 'normal' time, too.

'I found the hospice scary at first,' she explained. 'There were a lot of profoundly sick children there; I was really only used to my sister. But I loved being able to have my mum and dad to myself during the times when Isobel stayed there for respite.'

Chloe has very fond memories of time spent at the hospice – playing in the garden, surrounded by toys, and trips to the ice rink with her parents. Her face lit up when she told me about her time with the hospice play therapist; it was clear that this had been a positive experience for her.

'She came to the house to see me for quite a few visits,' she recalled. 'It was just time for me. I didn't need to talk to anyone else or share my time with anyone else. Our sessions together were just for me and that was a good feeling.'

Eventually, as Isobel's health stabilised, her tracheostomy was removed and she spent less time in hospital, and the support from the hospice ended. This can happen – no one really knows how a child will respond and develop. There were even a few fleeting months in Daisy's life when I wondered if she really needed the hospice. We met many families through the hospice who would 'graduate' from it. It was something to be celebrated: they had been given a lifeline of support when their child was at their sickest, but sometimes children do stabilise. It doesn't mean Isobel will be cured; it just means that she's no longer as sick as she was. Her transplanted liver is working well, she goes to school, eats and walks independently, and talks non-stop!

But while Isobel's health is now stable and hospital admissions are a very rare occurrence, Chloe still lives with the anxiety and trauma of those early years.

'A few years ago, Isobel needed to have some teeth out under general anaesthetic,' she told me. 'I was a mess. I asked my teacher if I could go home; I couldn't focus. I was terrified that something would happen to my sister.'

She readily admits that she's overly protective of her sister. 'In my head, I imagine when I have a house, there'll be an annexe for Isobel and I can pay her to help look after my kids and never leave the house without me. I don't want her to live anywhere apart from with Mum and Dad or me.'

Chloe missed out on having a 'normal' sibling relationship; she became a young carer as soon as Isobel was born. It shaped her childhood, and it continues to shape her adult life as she reflects back on her experiences.

If she could go back, what would she say to the professionals caring for her sister?

'Don't lose sight of the siblings,' she told me. 'I wasn't that much into siblings' groups or hanging around in the hospital playroom with the other kids. We get forgotten about; no one quite knows what to do about us, but it impacts our lives, too – our childhood.'

As I said to Daisy's social worker – my children only get one shot at childhood here. It's not just about Daisy.

Much of what Chloe told me is echoed in my daughter Xanthe's experience, too.

Xanthe's story

My elder daughter, Xanthe, is the reason Daisy got her name. She was supposed to be called Ophelia Rose, but our feisty five-year-old, beside herself that the gender balance had been equalled out in the family, insisted that her baby sister should be called Daisy Rose.

'I don't remember much about Daisy's early days in hospital,' she told me. 'I was just ecstatic to have a sister. I remember planning all the special things we could do together. I honestly don't remember any concern or upset. I was just so happy that there was this little baby girl in our family.'

I've got a wonderful picture of Xanthe in the neonatal unit, sitting with Daisy in her arms and holding up the syringe that's attached to her nasogastric tube as a nurse administers her feed. Xanthe took it in her stride; she saw her sister, not her sister's problems.

As Xanthe got older and it became obvious that Daisy was different from other babies, she became very careful about telling people what was going on. Not because she wanted to hide what was happening, but because, as she told me, 'this was my story and my life'.

It was clear in talking to her that she didn't want to be defined by what was happening at home.

'I think at primary school it was easier,' she told me, 'because my friends knew Daisy from day one, and they knew about my life. But once I went to secondary school, I was very careful who I decided to tell about what was happening. It was important that my friends didn't treat my sister differently – she was my sister at the end of the day – so I had to be careful who I allowed to see my life at home.'

There's a real sense of wanting to protect her sister when Xanthe speaks. Just in the same way Chloe feels that sense of responsibility. Like so many siblings of children with complex needs, Xanthe feels she had to grow up very quickly. She felt a weight of responsibility, both as a young carer but also because she did not want to add to my stresses. That hit hard. I really tried to find a balance between being open and honest about Daisy's condition and prognosis and ensuring my children had a happy childhood. I didn't want them to worry. But that was inescapable.

'When I was little, I couldn't make sense of it,' Xanthe told me. 'I would become irritated if one of my parents was away. I just wanted us all to be at home together. But as I grew up, I felt more of a sense of what was happening and the stress my parents were under. My anger turned to empathy,' she continued, 'as I realised what they were dealing with. And I tried not to add to that or make things worse for them.'

There is no sense of resentment towards Daisy, just a gradual adjustment and sadness.

'In the early years, I didn't really worry about what the future would hold for Daisy,' Xanthe explained. 'I just enjoyed being with her and having a sister. I think as I got older, I realised that it was not normal for a sister to be in and out of hospital and to need so much medical support. But it was all we ever knew of life with Daisy. I think when she started to have seizures and deteriorated, that's when I really knew that there would be a day when she wouldn't be here any more. I mentally prepared myself that there would be a day when she didn't come home from hospital.'

That's a tough one for a mum to hear. It's bittersweet in many ways. Andy and I had tried to be open and realistic, not give false hope or hide the truth. Our children, like us, lived daily with the burden of knowing that one day Daisy would die.

Thank goodness for our hospice. Not only did they support Daisy with respite, but they played a really important role in all my children's lives. It's wonderful to hear how important the experience of hospice support was for both Chloe and Xanthe.

'To me, the hospice was one of my favourite things ever,' Xanthe told me. 'I actually felt privileged to be able to go to such a brilliant place. The happiest memories of my childhood are of time spent there with my family.'

I cannot begin to imagine how differently things would have turned out if Ruth had not made that referral to the hospice when Daisy was a few months old. I knew that for my children it was one of their favourite places, but it was hearing Xanthe speak so animatedly about how important the stays at the hospice were to her that really made it hit home.

My children had to grow up so quickly. They had to become independent and self-reliant from an early age. And all the while knowing that their sister, whom they adored, was going to die.

I think they all built up armour to protect themselves. Just like Chloe, the impact of what they saw, heard and experienced runs deep.

It's important that professionals see the sick child as a person within a family unit, yet, all too often, support and care is ruled by budgets. There was a budget to get Daisy to school but no help to get my other children to school while I was getting Daisy sorted. With no close family nearby, I relied on a network of friends to help out. My children adored Daisy – she was the centre of their world, and they have many happy memories of time spent with her – but each of them has also had their own issues. My two boys were diagnosed late with forms of autism. I just didn't spot it, and their school put their behaviour down to anxiety and worry about what was going on at home. All three of my children have needed therapeutic input tailored to their needs, which inevitably I had to pay for because there was simply nothing suitable available on the NHS.

My kids, now young adults like Chloe, have seen and experienced things that no parent ever wants for their child. They were kept awake by Daisy screaming in pain at night. They also had to put up with carers and nurses always being in the house, reassuring their friends when Daisy had a massive tonic-clonic seizure

ANYTHING FOR MY CHILD

in the middle of their birthday party, their parents rarely being at home at the same time, our short tempers from lack of sleep and constant stress, cancelled plans, lives spent in hospital playrooms, not knowing if their sister would still be at home when they woke up in the morning or blue-lighted back into hospital overnight... The list goes on.

My kids just wanted to fit in, not stand out, yet being siblings of a disabled sister with complex health needs made this impossible. Like Chloe, their weekends were often spent in hospital. The hospice was a welcome respite for us all, but they found it difficult to explain to school friends why they got to stay at this amazing place full of toys and fun every now and then.

I remember being so excited when Daisy got her first wheelchair. She learned very quickly to wheel herself independently. I loved that she'd transitioned from her special needs stroller into a chair that gave her a bit more independence. Theo, my eldest, hated it, however. 'Now she really looks disabled, and I don't want people staring at her,' he told me.

The ripples of care run far and wide. Relationships break down and friendships are lost. Parents live in a state of hypervigilance. I felt I was constantly trying to keep multiple plates spinning, keeping everyone happy and on an even keel, trying desperately just to be Mum and not a nurse, or carer or advocate. There were times when I really resented the carers who came in to help during the daytime. They were having fun with Daisy while I was busy cleaning the house, ordering the medical ancillaries I needed to manage Daisy's TPN, catching up with the shopping or helping my other kids with their homework. Times to just be a parent, let alone a wife and partner, were few and far between. And after that, there was just minimal time for me.

In focusing on our children's health, Andy and I neglected our own needs. We tried hard to make time for each other and catch up, but this was always dictated by Daisy's health and needs. We felt permanently exhausted. It's only in hindsight that I realise how tired I was.

Andy had depression. He'd been diagnosed with it just after my father died when our first two children were three and one. He took daily medication prescribed by our GP. Work was how he managed it. It gave him routine, focus and purpose.

Research has shown higher incidence rates of common and serious physical and mental health problems and death in mothers of children with a life-limiting condition.[1] In fact, it recommends that there may be a role to play by paediatric teams in supporting or signposting mothers of complex children to other services to support their own physical or mental health needs:

> These mothers will have many more contacts with paediatric healthcare providers than with their own healthcare provider, and there may be a role of paediatric providers in providing support or signposting to appropriate services. Family-centred care is an approach that has highlighted the importance of the family unit when providing health services to children with chronic conditions or disabilities, but the implementation of this model of care has been limited.

But even if this support had been in place, it would have missed the huge and unexpected shockwave that hit our family in late 2014.

---

1   Fraser, L.K., Murtagh, F.E., Aldridge, J., Sheldon, T., Gilbody, S. and Hewitt, C. (2021) 'Health of mothers of children with a life-limiting condition: A comparative cohort study.' *Archives of Disease in Childhood 106*, 10, 987–993.

CHAPTER 11

Caring for the Carers

ANDY BEGAN TO LOSE WEIGHT. It was unexplained and rapid. He then became symptomatic – bleeding from his bottom, abdominal pain, vomiting. By November, he had been diagnosed with stage four, incurable colorectal cancer. In hindsight, the warning signs were there. He was tired and breathless a lot, he just had no energy. But we just put it down to getting older – he was now 51 – and our ridiculous workload, also balanced with his career. By the time he was diagnosed he was found to be acutely anaemic and seriously deficient in Vitamin D.

The cancer, as it stood, was inoperable. He needed chemotherapy and targeted radiotherapy to see if the tumours could shrink enough to make the prospect of surgery a possibility.

His oncologist told me, 'Supporting your husband through this will bring you to your knees.' I laughed. I was already staring over the edge of the abyss, living knowing my child was going to die before she reached adulthood.

The fact that I was now caring for a very sick husband and daughter seemed to galvanise services into action. Suddenly, our care package was increased, including regular funded respite stays at a residential centre that was able to care for children with Daisy's complexity.

Why did it need my husband's cancer diagnosis for this to happen? What if we had received this support before he became ill? Would we have noticed his symptoms earlier? Would it have reduced the state of constant hypervigilance that we lived in that maybe (I just postulate here) contributed to the cancer?

Andy lived for a year after his diagnosis. However, despite aggressive chemotherapy and experimental radiotherapy, his tumours remained inoperable. He developed radiation-induced liver damage and the break from chemo to allow his liver to recover caused the cancer to run haywire. A week before Daisy's 11th birthday, he came home from hospital to die. The children's hospice opened up their emergency bed, and as Daisy left the house with a nurse, Andy mustered up all the remaining strength he had left to say goodbye to her. It was the last word he said; within a few hours, knowing that Daisy was safe in the hospice and our other children were nearby, he took his final breaths and died.

We met when I was 20, at university. I was now a widowed single parent of four children under the age of 18. I was caring for a very sick little girl and three grieving siblings, two of whom were neurodiverse. I had no family nearby. I was on my own. At least we had our carers and nurses helping us out, or so I thought.

Within a few weeks of Andy's funeral, I was contacted by our community nursing team. There had been a request to review the package of care that was in place. It was very expensive and had been put together to support me while Andy was ill. The implication was that now I was no longer caring for my sick husband, I could focus on my sick child and didn't need so much extra help.

If Andy's diagnosis hadn't brought me to my knees, the news that the lifeline of support, the news that the ability to be able to sleep at night, knowing a nurse was keeping Daisy safe, was about to be taken away from me certainly did.

It shouldn't be a surprise that parents end up using combative language – fighting for support becomes the norm. The hopes and dreams we have for our family have been shattered; our children enter adulthood reflecting on a childhood that is so different from their peers. Memories for them are of time in hospital, interspersed with meetings with celebrities or trips to Disney. There is no predictability in our lives, apart from the predictability that plans will change.

The closest we had to holistic family support was the hospice. As Chloe recalled, the support her family received from the hospice is an important part of her childhood memory – the space to just talk given to her through play therapy that she still remembers well over a decade later, a chance just to have her parents to herself.

I know that time spent at the hospice was the happiest of times for my children. They could let their guard down without fear of anyone judging or watching. We were incredibly lucky, though: we have a brilliant children's hospice nearby and we had a consultant who referred us very early on. Not every family gets that sort of support. Not every sibling gets the chance to talk or to just get time with their parents.

If Xanthe and Chloe are still processing the impact of growing up as a young carer, as the sibling of a child who is medically complex and life-limited, despite having support as children, what must it be like for all those other siblings who, because of where they live, have missed out on support?

Marriages break down, family units fall apart, and the pressure on the parents caring for medically complex children is immense. It's only now, as I look back, that I realise how much I've been through. It took a minor car accident when I was running on empty for my GP to point out that I was suffering from post-traumatic stress disorder (PTSD).

We have no choice: we have to keep going, day in, day out, one foot in front of the other. We ignore our health, and we burn ourselves out trying to keep all of the plates spinning.

And we are alone. Because there are no 24-hour services to support us, we're there at home, trying to work out whether it's appropriate to give another dose of pain meds or call an ambulance.

My situation is extreme. Never in a million years did I see Andy's cancer coming, that I would be left alone to care for our daughter, our children. But life happens, and families need to feel supported; they need to feel cared for – not that they are justifying every penny.

As I pointed out time and time again, we are not talking long-term here...but for our family, it's a lifetime.

◇ CHAPTER 12 ◇

Palliative Care Is Not Giving Up

T HERE ARE MANY MOMENTS ETCHED IN MY MEMORY as I look back on my life as Daisy's mum: being told at eight weeks' pregnant that there was a one-in-four chance that she had Down's syndrome, the day I left my office and swung by the antenatal clinic to see if a midwife was around as 'things just didn't feel right' (it was to be the last day I ever worked full-time in an office), Daisy's birth, her diagnosis, the night her first ever bag of TPN was hung up (it was Bonfire Night and this moment was heralded with the sound of fireworks being let off around London)...surgeries, referrals and conversations. Each of them marked a waypoint on our journey with Daisy.

There's one that stands out as the moment, in hindsight, when the long and slow decline to end of life really began. The day in 2013 when Daisy had her first epileptic seizure.

I'd been worried about Daisy's neurology for a while. She seemed to have absence seizures where she was in her own world. We had also had a couple of episodes where she had not been able to breathe that were put down to laryngeal spasms. Those had been scary enough – nothing, though, in comparison to the moment when, after a busy day visiting friends, I was getting Daisy ready for bed and preparing her TPN infusion while Andy was making dinner in the kitchen.

Daisy could still walk at that point and was pottering around her room. The next moment, she let out a scream, became very still, then dropped to the floor, convulsing violently, her face blue from lack of oxygen.

I had just witnessed a classic tonic-clonic seizure, but I did not know it at the time. I thought she was dying. 'This is it,' I thought. 'This is how it ends.'

She was blue-lighted to our local hospital. They stabilised her. Within a few hours, we were home again. And that was how the unwelcome visitor came to our home. Epilepsy really did mark the beginning of the end. I don't know if there was a direct correlation, but she began to lose skills: within months walking was no longer possible; her language, minimal as it was, began to deteriorate; her behaviour began to become more and challenging as she hit out at nurses and carers and anyone who dared to get too close...

Over the next few years, compounded by Andy's cancer diagnosis, treatment and death, I witnessed the loss of 'Daisy'. The long, slow decline really heightened our awareness of what was important for her, what constituted an acceptable quality of life and how far we would be prepared to go in achieving this for her.

We were fortunate because these discussions had begun a couple of years previously. We had been referred to the children's palliative care team at Great Ormond Street Hospital during a long hospital stay, where it became clear that there were very few options on the table for Daisy. We always knew she would not be cured, but it was evident that she was always going to be dependent on TPN. Other things had started to go wrong: her bladder did not function properly, and more and more of her bowel was being removed.

'I don't want to leave a stone unturned,' I had told Daisy's doctors. 'I want to make sure that, at the end, I explored all options.'

Those options had included discussions about a multivisceral transplant. We had seen other children go through this surgery, to replace stomach, small bowel, pancreas and sometimes liver with transplanted organs in one procedure. We knew it would never be an option for Daisy, but we wanted to bring it up, to ensure that we had the conversation, so that we could at least say we discussed it as an option.

Children with Costello syndrome have a 15 per cent higher risk than a typical child of developing malignancies. We knew that anti-rejection drugs post-transplant would increase her chance of developing cancer, and we knew that she would still have Costello syndrome regardless. We also knew that there was a risk that she could die in surgery and that the surgery might not even help her get off TPN. It was not a risk that we wanted to explore further.

The biggest issue we faced was how to manage Daisy's complex pain effectively. A professor of gastroenterology, visiting from a specialist children's hospital in Cincinnati, came to review Daisy when she was an inpatient one day. He explained to me in lay terms how rather than becoming more tolerant to pain, children with complex and chronic pain can actually feel it more intensely.

'It's like beating a pathway through the jungle,' he explained. 'The more you use the pathway, the easier it is to navigate your way through the undergrowth and the quicker you reach your destination.'

Apparently, it's the same with pain pathways. With constant pain, the neurons become 'hypervigilant' and more efficient at carrying messages to the brain. In other words, the constant pain meant that Daisy felt it more intensely. There is no such thing as 'building up tolerance to pain' – that's just a myth, according to the professor.

And, of course, managing a child with such chronic pain is immensely difficult.

We were struggling to find ways to manage her pain safely at home. Daisy's colon had been removed as this was one source of pain, and she had an ileostomy. Her bladder pain was very difficult to manage; she would scream out at night with horrific bladder spasms, and we felt so helpless.

That's when we were referred to the hospital palliative care team.

We were lucky, first of all to be under a hospital that has a paediatric palliative care team and also to have been referred to the team by a consultant with the foresight to involve them at an early stage. It was another important tipping point for Daisy. Over and over, doctors, nurses and professionals ask me how they should broach difficult conversations with families, how should they prepare parents for the fact that their child is going to die in order to discuss their wishes.

'Begin those conversations early,' I always respond. 'Not when there is a crisis. And couch them in terms of living, not dying; quality of life, not end of life'.

I spoke recently to a palliative consultant in another hospital. 'Even our own colleagues call us the grim reaper,' she told me. 'We're the last to be called, when everyone else has run out of options and nothing more can be done.'

If anything, it's too late then; it's too late to build up trust, to have difficult conversations to discuss options. When Andy had cancer, the palliative consultant was introduced at the very end of his life, when the oncologist told us there was nothing more they could do, that the only option was palliative care. At that point, our conversations were around whether he wanted to die at home or at the hospice.

Being introduced to paediatric palliative care early gave us an important opportunity to discuss many issues, to ask questions, but, most importantly, to focus on Daisy's quality of life. It was clear she was not at the end of life, but that early referral meant we had time to discuss what was important for Daisy and to make plans. When Andy died and Daisy was at the end of life, I knew what we had both wanted for her, what was important. I felt in control because I had prepared for that moment for a long time.

Keeping Daisy out of hospital was always our priority. Our palliative consultant worked with our hospice to develop a pain management regimen for her so that we had levels of escalation at home. She spent a few days in the hospice so that the team could work out the best regimen to help her, and our end result was a plan that would put control back in our hands when we had felt so helpless in managing Daisy's pain.

At last, we felt that we had someone in our corner. The palliative team crossed the different specialities and, more importantly, they came into our world. Sometimes Daisy's consultant would visit us at home or if she was staying at the hospice; they would come along to big hospital appointments with the intestinal failure team. If Daisy was an inpatient, then a team member would visit regularly. If there was a multi-disciplinary meeting, then they would attend.

We began to have those difficult conversations, in what felt like a place of safety.

How far did we want to go in Daisy's care? Andy and I agreed that if it came to the point that Daisy would need a tracheostomy to breathe, then we would not go down that route. By that stage, she had five different tubes and stomas keeping her alive: a double-lumen central venous catheter taped to her chest and permanently connected to a pump, drip-feeding her precious TPN fluids; a gastrostomy which drained bile from her stomach into a bag; a jejunostomy into her small intestine for very small volumes of drugs that could not be given intravenously; an ileostomy stoma where her colon had been removed; and a Mitrofanoff stoma – a specialist tract into her bladder formed from her appendix, which had a catheter permanently inserted into it that was connected to a urine bag. Daisy was mobile (in her wheelchair), and she could sit up independently. It was enough to be able to try to be a little girl with all of this going on, we reasoned; by the time she needed a tracheostomy, her quality of life, of the life that she knew, would have been so severely depleted that we felt it would be a step too far.

Quality of life. What does that mean? How do you measure it? What constitutes an acceptable quality of life?

That's the reason for this book. It's what I have tried to explore when I interviewed parents, family members and professionals. And as with every ethical dilemma, there are no clear answers, no right and wrong; there are just difficult decisions.

When you are the parent of a child with complex medical needs, the pressure to make the right decision, to do the right thing as their advocate, is huge.

If you had read Daisy's notes at that time – with all those ostomies, the drug chart that extended to several pages, the multi-focal epilepsy that was not fully controlled despite a cocktail of drugs, the pain, the deteriorating heart function, the loss of skills – you would think that Daisy had a very poor quality of life. To an outsider, it could appear that way. But because we lived with Daisy 24/7, we understood the subtleties, the important things, the things that Daisy wanted us to know. It was always very simple for Daisy, as for us: the little things were in fact the big things. All she wanted to do was to try to get to school as often as possible, to spend time with her siblings, to play with her beloved dog, Pluto. That's what we needed to focus on. Daisy drew every day from reserves; she channelled strength to just get through the day and enjoy her life. We did everything in our power to make sure that she was able to be a little girl, to stay out of hospital and to be at home.

'We have a window with Daisy,' I told the palliative consultant. 'We will know when that window begins to narrow that we are nearing the end. But while we have a window, we will do whatever we can to give her the best possible quality of live we can.'

That's how we measured every medical decision and plan: if the window was open, if Daisy was still able to do the things she loved and engage in family life, then we would agree to whatever treatment was necessary to enable that.

The time Andy was undergoing chemotherapy coincided with some big decisions about whether Daisy should have yet another complicated and risky surgery. Her bladder was causing more and more problems. Now that all of her large bowel, her rectum and a section of small bowel had been removed, much of her pain was focused on her bladder (I was told that this was not a surprise given the disordered neuropathy of both her bowel and bladder). She was in extreme pain and the Mitrofanoff stoma, the special tract that enabled us to pass a catheter from her tummy directly into her bladder, was narrowing and becoming less efficient. She was on two litres of TPN fluid every 24 hours and often needed additional fluids to correct electrolyte imbalances. This meant that we could not empty her bladder fully, increasing her risk of infection (her bladder was permanently colonised with various bugs at this stage), or damage to her kidneys. And the pain was unbearable for her.

The urology surgeon was keen to go in and try to find a better solution; however, there was disagreement among the other members of Daisy's team – including the surgeon who had previously operated on her and her intestinal failure team. I found out afterwards that Daisy's case was discussed at the hospital's clinical ethics committee.

While I didn't want Daisy to go through yet another very long and complex surgery, I also did not want her to be in so much pain, and there was also her dignity. While her catheter had worked, Daisy had been able to wear 'big girl knickers'; her urine and faeces drained into bags, and she didn't need nappies. This had made her very, very happy. Having to once more revert to nappies as her bladder failed caused her much distress, and she would frequently rip them off and throw them over the side of the bed in anger.

The operation took place. We took the view that the chance of being able to help Daisy's pain outweighed the very real and present risk that she could die in surgery. It was probably the most heavily discussed and debated procedure that she had been through. The stress of making the decision was immense, compounded by the fact that Andy was also very ill, the brutal chemotherapy taking its toll on his health. But we also knew that the window had not closed for Daisy yet, that while she was clearly on a downward trajectory, she was not at the end of life, and we owed it to her to do everything possible to make whatever time she had left with us matter, to give quality to her life.

As we accompanied Daisy to theatre, she made the Makaton sign for 'home'. That was all she wanted.

This surgery took place around 14 months before Daisy's death, but it removed some of the most excruciating pain and gave her back some dignity during that time.

Having a good relationship with our palliative team helped us make these decisions and helped us get clarity. They didn't tell us what to do, but they supported us, gave us options, helped us see what was possible and helped us to support Daisy's wish to be at home with her family, her siblings and her dog. For us, working with palliative care was not about giving up: it was about living.

The words 'palliative care' did not scare us. We knew that Daisy would tell us when it was time, when the window was closing. I relied on my instinct that we could discuss plans and options, but all of those were fluid: we would know in the end. We accepted very early on that Daisy would die, but that she would call the shots on when and how. We just needed to be prepared to know how to support that.

When I interviewed Gemma, she was similarly logical. She has spent her nursing career in paediatric palliative care and knows what those on the outside refuse to see: that sometimes children die.

'We were referred to the palliative care team after Zoe's cardiac arrest,' she told me, 'when it was decided once and for all that she could not have a transplant. I know that it didn't mean she was dying, but I understood that there were no more treatment options that could potentially either extend her life or even make her better. I'd got my head around that quite a while ago, to be honest – it was just hearing it out loud. It was really upsetting. And I remember sobbing on the phone to my mum.'

Gemma takes reassurance from the support of the palliative care team; they are the people who are on the end of the phone, who know what is going on with Zoe, the team helping to ensure that Zoe maximises her quality of life.

It's a sad, sad fact of life that children do die before they reach adulthood. Knowing and accepting that fact sharpens the mind on living every single moment, and for us, and for Gemma, good palliative care support helps achieve this.

For many people, the words 'palliative care' conjure up fear. About imminent death, about giving up. It's couched in a negative light: there is no more that can be done.

Maybe there needs to be a rebranding of the speciality. If palliative consultants struggle to be supported by their own colleagues, to be involved earlier, then no wonder parents see a referral to the palliative team as a negative last step before death.

Saira's story[1]

Saira's daughter Samara was deprived of oxygen at birth, which resulted in severe brain damage. By the time she was three, Samara had developed epilepsy, experiencing seizure after seizure. Saira was now a single parent, bringing up her precious and much-loved daughter on her own, living with her widowed father for support and help. Brain surgery to try to control the debilitating seizures was unsuccessful; Saira was told that there was nothing more that could be done for her daughter and all further care would be aimed at trying to manage Samara's symptoms.

I met Saira at a family day at Daisy's hospice. By this time, Samara was already in her early teens. Saira's life revolves around her daughter, often at the sacrifice of her own health and emotional needs. Samara wants for nothing; she is, as Saira frequently tells me, a true princess.

'The biggest thing I fear, the thing that makes me the most anxious, is the thought of life without my beloved daughter,' Saira told me in an emotional conversation. 'I cannot bear to think of her dying, but I also cannot bear to think of her suffering.'

Which is why Saira has been discussing and preparing for the thing she most dreads since Samara turned 14. Samara's health has been in a steady decline; she now needs non-invasive ventilation via a CPAP mask every night and often, when she is unwell, during the day. Her seizures are much worse, and she often has frequent periods of status epilepticus, a life-threatening condition where she experiences almost constant seizure activity in her brain.

A simple cold can trigger a dangerous chest infection and hospital admission. It was one of these episodes a few years ago that really brought home to me the fine line Saira walks with Samara's health.

'Her CPAP was on maximum pressure, and yet Sammy was still working hard,' Saira told me. 'I spoke to the respiratory consultant about tracheostomy, but he did not think that it was a viable option

---

1   Name changed.

– he felt that it would not be fair on her. I just did not know where to turn.'

It's clear how painful it is to even think about her daughter's death, but working closely with a palliative consultant, Saira has made plans and had the discussions that she hates but knows she needs to have. It's clear how much Samara's respiratory doctor and palliative consultant care for and understand Saira's situation. With their careful support and constant guidance, Saira has been able to clearly develop a plan for her daughter's care and support as she edges ever closer to end of life.

'I need to keep her at home,' Saira told me. 'I need to avoid hospital at all costs; I want my daughter to die at home, and any hospital visit risks that not happening.'

So everything is focused on supporting Saira and Samara to stay at home. Samara's feeding tube has to be changed under general anaesthetic and it's managed as a day case. Community nurse support means that any intravenous antibiotics are given at home, and there are plans in place for any escalations of care.

'I have worked with our palliative consultant and the rest of Sammy's team to discuss lots of different scenarios. I've allowed myself to go there so I can think about what would be best for her when it comes to the end,' Saira told me. 'We know that her breathing is getting worse, her seizures are getting worse; we know that this may be the last year with her.'

One of the scenarios she has discussed is what happens to Samara after she dies; it's important to Saira that she remains in her home until the funeral.

'But if she dies at home and our GP has not seen her that month, I don't want to risk a post-mortem,' Saira told me, 'so I now have an arrangement with them that they facetime me every four weeks so that they can see Sammy.'

In other words, despite the fact that Samara's death will not be unexpected, ensuring that she's seen by her GP every few weeks means that there will be a minimal risk of a post-mortem being required by a coroner.

Years of careful communication, patience and planning have brought Saira to this point. She cannot bear to think of her daughter dying, but she knows there is nothing she can do to prevent it, and the most important thing is to ensure that she does not suffer. She has planned and discussed every possible scenario with Samara's palliative team, taking herself through the pain of facing the inevitable in order to ensure that when Sammy chooses her time, her death will be a good death at home, with her devoted mum beside her.

Fathers Care, Too

W HAT IS IT LIKE TO BE A FATHER of a medically complex child? I'm acutely aware that my focus has been through the eyes of mothers so far. There's little if any detailed research on the impact on fathers, and in not discussing it and exploring Andy's experiences as Daisy's father, I'm missing a whole other part of the story.

I guess because Andy is dead, I've become entrenched in my own lived experience. I wish I could ask him what it was like, but I only have my own memories to go on.

I've already mentioned that Andy suffered from depression. He took medication for it and this helped him a lot. When Daisy was born, his depression took a downturn. He initially had trouble adapting to the sudden change in our lives that had taken place with her early arrival and the subsequent talk of genetic conditions and a shortened lifespan. He struggled with the uncertainties that we were now facing about our future and what might lie ahead.

I remember that there were times during Daisy's two-month stay in the neonatal unit when he couldn't face coming to visit. Once I was discharged from the hospital following my caesarean delivery, I would travel back and forth to the neonatal unit on a daily basis. I needed the routine and structure. Expressing milk, waiting for the ward round, managing Daisy's care, just trying to be there as much as possible for my baby until she was well enough to come home. Andy had gone back to work by this time, and our older children were back at school or with their childminder.

Once Daisy came home, this division of labour continued. The children's half-term holiday fell a week later, and Andy took the three older children away to France, leaving me with Daisy. I had thought it was a good idea at the time, but it was awful. Daisy wouldn't sleep, and I struggled to get enough nutrition into her. She cried all the time and was becoming increasingly dehydrated and unsettled. By the time Andy returned home, I was on my knees, desperate for some adult conversation and someone to help carry the load as I worried about our baby.

I remember our GP telling me to be careful not to fall into a dynamic where I took the lead in caring for Daisy, but I did, or rather we did. I was on maternity leave, and it was becoming increasingly clear that returning to work was not going to be an option. Most of my maternity leave had been spent in hospital with Daisy or at outpatient appointments, and there was no sign of that changing, which would make managing a full-time career pretty tricky. So although I was the major wage earner in our relationship, I handed in my notice and became a full-time mother and carer, something that I had never intended to do. I had always prided myself on building my career. My hope had been to reduce my work hours at some stage; I had never entertained the thought of not working at all.

But as far as I was concerned, Daisy needed me, and I needed to be there not just for her but for our entire family. I also felt that it was vital for Andy's mental health that he had the structure and routine of work. I knew that I would not have been able to manage juggling a career with Daisy's ever-increasing complexity. We did not discuss this; it just happened. With hindsight, I regret not having the conversation, and I guess I'm angry at the assumption that I would sacrifice my career to be the main carer. It didn't occur to me to approach my employer to discuss options or whether my job could be held open until I knew what was happening. I didn't go back to work, and Andy built his career. But there were times when

I really resented him for his life outside our complicated home life. I missed being with other people. I missed people thanking me for doing a good job. I was lonely and isolated, and I didn't know who I was any more. I was no longer Stephanie, Head of Marketing; I was Daisy's mum, Andy's wife or just plain Mum...

There's still a gender imbalance in caring. The majority of carers are women, and when it comes to caring for a child with medical complexity, the role of main carer falls very much at the feet of the mother. I remember the evenings on the gastro ward in Great Ormond Street Hospital. The day staff had gone home, the visitors had gone, and it was mostly mothers staying over with their children. I remember one of the Muslim mothers on the ward at the time feeling safe enough to remove her hijab on some evenings because everyone on the ward was female or a child.

Andy spent plenty of time in hospital as Daisy grew older, but the two of us had very different styles. I would sit balancing a microwave meal on my lap in the corner of Daisy's room, willing her to fall asleep so that I could close my eyes and switch off at last. I would put up all of Daisy's intravenous medications and drips when she was in hospital, whereas Andy relied on the nurses to come in and take over so that he could take some time out. Andy's not here to discuss this, but as I've been writing this book, I've reflected a lot on how we divided our roles during that time. Could he have done more? Should I have done less? There were plenty of occasions when he would go straight to work from the hospital. But at the same time, going home to our other children was not a rest for me; they had their own issues, and we were also going through the process of obtaining an autism diagnosis for our elder son.

There was also a marked difference in our communication styles with professionals. I would really try to be collaborative. I wanted our teams on our sides; I needed them to like us and want to work with us. Andy had a different approach, rooted in his expectations that they should be doing things for us. I tended to take the lead in conversations with clinicians; I'd bring Andy in when there were problems.

As a fellow mother caring for a child with complexity told me, 'Sometimes I just needed to bring in the testosterone to shake them all up; they would listen to him.'

Some parents I have spoken to have felt that the tone of the doctors changed when the father became involved in meetings. As one fellow Costello syndrome mother told me:

> I send Nic (my husband) when I can't get what I want done, or if I don't feel like arguing. I argued for 18 months that something was wrong with the baby. I finally told Nic he had to take her. He got a referral for a sleep study that day and she was back on oxygen (which is exactly what I said she needed) within weeks.

It can feel a little like institutionalised sexism on behalf of the clinicians at times – the mum is the one who is involved on a day-to-day basis whereas the father could be more detached and even less emotional.[1]

I guess because I was seeing the clinicians more regularly, I was careful to manage our relationships, whereas Andy would push back and question if he felt things weren't being done properly or happening quickly enough. There were definitely times when this was needed. Once, a doctor came in to examine Daisy on the ward. He did so without washing his hands, and Andy immediately jumped in, shouting at him to stop. Daisy was MRSA-positive at the time; she'd probably contracted the superbug as a result of someone else not washing their hands and then examining her. Another time, he told a surgeon off for examining Daisy without asking her permission or talking to her. She was lying in bed, post-surgery, and he just came in and lifted her gown. 'Would you have leapt in and examined any other eight-year-old girl without asking her permission?' Andy demanded. He was right, and I was grateful that he was there to call those health professionals out.

The online groups, the social groups, the support networks

---

1   Although it seems a generalisation, many mothers have commented anecdotally about the change in tone from some clinicians when the child's father was part of a meeting.

– they are very much dominated by women caring for children with complexity. I know Andy really did not want to get involved in the everyday online chatter, and he definitely did not want to be part of any 'dad groups' that our hospice offered. He would lurk and comment to me occasionally, but I was the one that did all the online research, chatting to other mums, asking advice online.

I wanted to understand how other fathers managed the changed dynamic once they were a parent to a child with medical complexity. The name that immediately sprang to mind was Alan. He and his wife, Lucy, are parents to a teenage daughter, Ruby. We met many years ago when both of our girls were patients on the gastro ward at Great Ormond Street. I remember Alan making the journey from Lincolnshire to Andy's funeral and wearing an Arsenal shirt (Andy's favourite football club) in his honour. I was really touched by that gesture.

I gave him a call to find out more about his own journey as Ruby's father.

Alan's story

Alan's a successful journalist and football writer, but this career is very recent. When he and his wife, Lucy, found out they were expecting their first child, he was a 23-year-old recent graduate and about to start a role in the local council as a democratic officer.

Midway through the pregnancy, scans began to show that there might be a problem. The doctors thought their baby daughter had an ovarian cyst, and from that moment Lucy was monitored more closely, her care transferred to a larger maternity centre further away from their home town. It was only after Ruby was born that it became clear that she didn't have an ovarian cyst but rather a problem with her bladder which was oversized and retaining too much urine.

'I'd only started my new job a week before,' Alan told me. 'My colleagues didn't know anything about what was going on with

Ruby. I was given three days' paternity leave, but fortunately, as she was born on Good Friday, I ended up with a bit more time off.'

Ruby was in hospital for about nine days. When she came home, she had a supra-pubic catheter to drain the urine from her bladder, and the couple were taught how to manage the dressings and keep it clean. But over the following weeks, it was clear that there was more going on with their baby beyond an enlarged bladder, and she began spending more and more time in hospital as doctors investigated problems that were emerging with her bowel function.

'I couldn't drive at that time,' Alan told me, 'so I would catch the train after work to go to Nottingham to see Lucy and Ruby. We just went with the flow; we didn't question the doctors. We didn't have friends with children, let alone friends with children with medical problems, so we just trusted that the doctors would find the answers and fix our daughter.'

Eventually, the family were referred to Great Ormond Street Hospital, and Ruby was found to have chronic intestinal pseudo-obstruction (which they now know is caused, in Ruby's case, by a genetic mutation). She began TPN and also had surgery to form an ileostomy stoma, which the doctors hoped would decompress her bowel.

The couple were taught how to manage Ruby's TPN and care for her stoma, making trips to London and to Nottingham on the train, and trying to manage at home.

After he had used up all of his annual leave within the first three months of the financial year, Alan's boss suggested he might want to have a think about his priorities. Alan resigned and breathed a sigh of relief.

The couple wondered how they were going to cope financially. 'I signed on for Jobseeker's Allowance because that's what I thought I had to do,' Alan told me. 'I would take a train back home from Great Ormond Street to attend interviews every week; no one was advising us about benefits or support or our rights – we just found this stuff out by talking to other people. We were so young. We didn't know about Disability Living Allowance and carer's benefits; we just were focused on trying to fix Ruby.'

But it was becoming clear that Ruby's condition was not fixable and that this was a long-term, medically complex condition they were dealing with. I wanted to know how the couple managed this.

'We realised that the doctors didn't have all the answers,' Alan told me, 'and they were trying different options, trying to find the answers. We fell into a routine: I would do a lot of the practical stuff while Lucy would do the research, contacting other families, finding out about potential drugs that might help and giving the information to the doctors.'

It sounded very familiar. I spent long evenings online trying to find answers, educating myself about Daisy's condition. Lucy, Alan's wife, was doing the same.

'The majority of the time, we just shared the care and everything that came with it, but it was Lucy that would question the doctors about possible treatments and present them with evidence she had found,' Alan told me. 'I got frustrated when we were in meetings with the doctors and they referred to me as "Dad", though,' he continued. 'I mean, we'd been under their care long-term, and they still didn't call me by my name.'

Things got worse for the family when Lucy had a fall and broke her leg badly. Alan then found himself caring for two people, in two different hospitals. 'I grew up very quickly in those years,' he told me. It was clear that over the years his confidence grew. The couple have worked out their routine for caring. Lucy takes the lead in meetings, whereas Alan is good with knowing Ruby's routines and regimens.

'We've got no qualms about correcting doctors or pushing back these days,' Alan told me, 'although Lucy does take the lead in challenging the doctors. In the beginning, we just accepted what we were told.'

Alan is now a successful journalist and football writer. I wanted to know how that had happened. 'Lucy's always been more supportive of me working than I have of myself!' he told me. 'I was careful not to take too much on at once and to build it up gradually, I just wanted to keep my CV ticking over with the aim of being able to get back to work at some point.'

It's clear that the couple are a good team. They communicate well and support each other, and there's no doubt that they had to grow up very quickly. 'We realised early on that we were in it for the long haul, and we had to make it work, for our marriage and for our family,' Alan told me.

'I now get frustrated when doctors don't take our own lived experience into account. When they don't realise what we've been through to get our daughter to this point.'

It was really interesting catching up with Alan. It was clear that they had worked hard to ensure that they were sharing the workload. I think, in the same way, Andy and I did what was right for us at the time. He needed to work, be with other people, but that put a big burden on me to manage the complexities of Daisy's care and to take the lead in dealing with the professionals.

It seems that this is a common story. Mothers take the lead in conversations with professionals, doing the research, learning the skills. And even where the father is very hands-on, this dynamic still continues.

In fact, there is evidence to show that fathers of children with medical complexity face problems in forming relationships with healthcare professionals. And this, coupled with role conflict in trying to maintain employment throughout their child's illness, can contribute to them feeling like observers in their child's care.[2]

The reality is that fathers who take the lead in caring for a child with medical complexity are still very much in the minority. I know lots of couples who share the workload. I know lots of couples whose relationship didn't withstand the stresses of parenting a medically complex child but who still co-parent. Some couples can find a

2   Fisher, V., Fraser, L. and Taylor, J. (2021) 'Experiences of fathers of children with a life-limited condition: A systematic review and qualitative synthesis.' *BMJ Supportive and Palliative Care 13*, 1. https://spcare.bmj.com/content/early/2021/06/28/bmjspcare-2021-003019

good balance which is respectful of the other's strengths as well as their wishes. But, on the whole, it is the mother who will tend to manage the majority of the care. Of course, there are same-sex partners who care for children with medical complexity, but the truth is that gender stereotypes around caring are still very much at the fore, and there are only rare examples of fathers being the main carer and driving the conversations and decisions.

Recently, I was introduced to Dougal. He's the main carer for his son, Oscar, and even he admits to being something of an anomaly.

Dougal's story

'Sometimes I go along to parent groups and I'm the only bloke there,' he told me. 'The other mums call me an "honorary mum" when they make plans for a night out and include me.'

Dougal had not planned to be the main carer for his son, but, as I know only too well, life has a funny way of changing your plans and throwing you into situations you just did not anticipate having to manage.

Dougal's son, Oscar, was still a baby when a failed hearing test led to more investigations. He was found to have seizure activity in his brain and was dual sensory impaired. It was clear that something was very wrong, and Dougal found himself having to juggle work in order to attend the ever-increasing list of hospital appointments with his wife and baby son.

'My wife didn't drive,' he explained, 'so I would have to take a day off work to drive them both to the hospital appointments.' It was also becoming clear to him that his wife was struggling to cope, both with the demands of adjusting to motherhood and the added concerns around her baby's increasingly apparent disabilities.

'I was doing shift work at the airport,' Dougal explained. 'I'd be up in the early hours doing Oscar's feed, then I'd be caring for him as soon as I got home. I took so much time off to attend hospital appointments that I had no annual leave left for us to have a holiday.' It all began to take its toll on the marriage and on his wife's mental health.

In the end, she decided to move back to live with her parents in another part of the country, leaving Dougal to care for Oscar.

'I was exhausted,' Dougal told me. 'I literally ended up collapsed on the floor of the kitchen, trying to juggle work, caring for Oscar, fighting for his school place and trying to save my marriage. It became evident that my wife had given me an ultimatum, to choose between her or Oscar. She would have preferred that he went into residential care, but there was no way I was going to allow that – he's my son, I'm not giving up on him.'

And that is how Dougal has ended up being the primary carer for his son. He has a team of carers to help at home, and Oscar, now 12, spends part of his time at a residential school, with the rest of the weekdays, weekends and school holidays at home with his dad, having what Dougal calls 'Dadventures'.

'The company I work for has been incredibly supportive,' Dougal told me. 'They said they would be as flexible as possible to make sure I could care for my son and still be able to work.'

I was really impressed with that. It means that Dougal has been able to balance caring for Oscar while not having to worry about money and letting his employer down. He's fortunate to have a good team of carers to support him in making it happen, too. Not everyone is able to make that work. We could barely get nurses to cover Daisy's school shifts; in the end, she was only able to go to school two days a week because there are simply not enough IV-trained nurses available to support families managing TPN at home.

But the understanding that a father can be the main carer is still not embedded in the system. Dougal recounted a time when he took Oscar to a hospital appointment with one of his carers, all of whom are women. 'The doctor immediately assumed the carer was Oscar's mum,' he told me. 'He did not expect me to be the one managing everything. Oscar's mum will now come to appointments with me occasionally, and the doctors still speak to her first, even though she doesn't live with us and is not involved in his care at all; she defers to me for all of this.'

It was lovely to speak to Dougal and refreshing to hear an example of a single dad taking the lead in caring for his child. There are other men out there doing the same, but the stereotype and expectation still remains when it comes to day-to-day care of a child with medical complexity, and the mother tends to take on the majority share.

Conflict and disagreement can change this dynamic, however. I felt I needed to be collaborative, to manage the relationships with professionals, to ensure that we had everyone on our side. I do recall Andy's approach being more combative – he expected things to happen, and he was a lot more direct in his communication with professionals.

CHAPTER 14

Fathers' Responses to Conflict

ARE THERE GENDER-BASED STEREOTYPES in how fathers manage conflict with healthcare professionals in comparison with mothers, or does it just boil down to the fact that we all respond and react differently?

Thomas Evans,[1] the young father of Alfie Evans, took the lead in speaking out publicly and disagreeing when his son's doctors recommended removing life-supporting treatment. He was very much the face and voice of the high-profile social media campaigns and media interviews, even sharing video footage of his son's final hours online.

His partner, Kate, Alfie's mother, was very much a figure in the background. In fact, in one of the final Court of Appeal hearings, the judge comments on this:

> Indeed, it is right to record that throughout the proceedings, and so far as one is concerned as a member of the public experiencing the press reporting from time to time in all other ways, whilst it has been the parents who have been opposing the actions of the hospital, it has been largely Alfie's father who has been at the forefront in displaying utter focus and tenacity in leading the campaign to reverse the decision of the judge.[2]

---

1   See Chapter 15 for more about the Alfie Evans case.
2   www.judiciary.uk/wp-content/uploads/2018/05/evans-v-alder-hey-appeal-judgment.pdf

Thomas's language online and in the media was combative, referring to his son as a warrior and a gladiator. For him, this was a battle against the system for his son's life, one that he had to win.

Thomas represented himself in the early case hearing at the family court, and the judge's report on this makes very moving reading (in this extract, F refers to Father):

> His core dilemma, from which he struggles to escape, is that whilst he recognises and understands fully that the weight of the evidence spells out the futility of Alfie's situation he is, as a father, unable to relinquish hope. This is to my mind entirely understandable. It is a facet of F's grief. In consequence, there is often a tension in the logic of his position. His personal conflict emerges in its starkest form in his attitude to the Alder Hey Hospital. Sometimes F is fulsome and generous in his tributes to the doctors and medical staff, on other occasions his criticisms are vituperative. This tension resonates in his approach to the medical evidence. It is, I think, no coincidence that F, whose primary position is that 'no stone should be left unturned', was resistant to the final MRI scan being undertaken. F, in my judgement, knew all too well, in the light of the earlier scans, what the latest MRI scan might reveal and, again for entirely understandable reasons, could not bear to confront it.[3]

Another, earlier, high-profile case caught my attention because the child at the centre, Jaymee Bowen,[4] was cared for solely by her father. Jaymee's birth mother had left the family home when Jaymee and her sister were still very young, and although her father, David, subsequently remarried, he was the central figure in the campaign for his daughter's treatment. A report in the *Independent* newspaper after Jaymee had died gives an interesting insight to his approach:

> Her father, David Bowen, a volatile and determined man, had decided she should be given the chance of life, however slim and whatever the human and financial cost. He committed himself

---

3   www.judiciary.uk/wp-content/uploads/2018/02/alder-hey-v-evans.pdf
4   See Chapter 17 for more about the Jaymee Bowen case.

to obtaining the treatment she needed, working night and day in libraries, telephoning experts around the world, cajoling and lying his way into their consulting rooms.[5]

I've struggled to find any research evidence on how fathers respond to conflict when disagreements arise with healthcare professionals caring for their child, but in these two cases the narrative was very much about fighting the system. Some insight to this behaviour may be gleaned from comments that David Bowen made at the time. He was driven partly by the realisation that he could not bear to see Jaymee die – to him, giving in was not on the agenda until every possible avenue of enquiry had been exhausted. 'They're good at trying to prepare you,' he said, 'the system will help you with anything to do with preparing yourself for the death of a child but it won't help you if you want to try and avoid that.'[6]

Do fathers struggle more with facing the fact that their child is going to die? Was this a factor driving the behaviour of Thomas Evans and David Bowen? What can healthcare professionals do to ensure that fathers feel involved in decisions about their child so that they don't feel their role is to lead the battle for their child's life when things don't go as they wished?

Is it about fight or flight?

One mother I interviewed (who wished to remain anonymous) told me that once it was clear her daughter was at the end stages of her life, her husband found it difficult to cope and spent less time at the hospice at his daughter's side. This had some echoes with Andy's initial lapse into depression when he found it difficult to spend time on the neonatal unit with Daisy.

Rosie remembers that when Matthias was becoming sicker and sicker, she told her husband, 'I love you, but our son needs me more now,' and she moved into his room to be close to him. Saira's husband could not cope with the fact that his longed-for daughter

5   Laurance, J. (1998) 'Child B: the truth about her last days.' *Independent*, 13 May. www.independent.co.uk/life-style/child-b-the-truth-about-her-last-days-1159951.html

6   Barclay, S. (1996) *Jaymee: The Story of Child B*. Viking.

was severely disabled; he walked away from the family unit and has never had anything to do with her since.

Does becoming a parent to a child with medical complexity trigger an extreme gender-based response among some parents? Is there unconscious bias in how some healthcare professionals treat mothers and fathers which reinforces perceived stereotypes? On the face of it, this seems to be the case.

What I do know, however, is that *both* parents need to be better supported in caring for their child so that they are not forced to fall into the stereotype of carer and provider through economic need. If only I had gone back to my employer and said, 'Look, I can't get back to work at the moment – my child needs me – but can we talk about ways that we could make it work if the possibility arises?' Would Dougal be able to cope as well as he has without the support of his employer over the years?

Every parent responds differently to the life changes that a medically complex child brings. It's a really lonely world; I know that and every parent I have spoken to has confirmed it. And this loneliness and feeling of disempowerment mean that we all find ways to reach out to amplify our voices or connect with a community of like-minded people going through the same.

That's where the internet, and social media, has added another level of complexity to how parents are able to communicate and shine a light on to their lived experience, as I explore in the next chapter.

CHAPTER 15

Generation Tagged

O NCE WE HAD CONFIRMATION that Daisy had the gene mutation that causes Costello syndrome, I decided to pluck up the courage to reach out to the CS Family Support Group. Like many similar rare disease groups, the CS group was the result of two parents finding each other online. By the time I stumbled across it, it had grown to a worldwide community of families, united by a sporadic mutation on the HRAS gene.

I enjoyed chatting to the other families and seeing pictures of their children. The physical similarities between them all were striking, but, as always, it seemed that the 'norm' for this rare disease was not Daisy's norm. It was really helpful to get tips on what to look out for to be able to share with Daisy's team, particularly as children with the syndrome were at increased risk of cancer and cardiac abnormalities. The latest research papers were always shared with the group by geneticists, so I was able to keep up to speed with what was happening and pass it on to doctors.

I also joined some online special needs support groups and began to make new friends in the local area. Having been thrust into this unknown world, forced to learn a new language, walk a new path, the internet gave me access to people who also understood what I was going through. Their journey was unique to them – some had a confirmed diagnosis for their child, some didn't – but the feelings of isolation, anxiety and helplessness were a common thread that united us all.

In the absence of any guidebook on how to navigate this new world of medical complexity, I also started following a few blogs written by other parent carers. It was good to be able to see into their worlds; their children were different to mine but the struggles were the same. I picked up so much useful information and was reassured to know that my feelings of helplessness were not unique to me and that there were other people I could reach out to.

Daisy was just three when I began to write my own blog. Initially, it was just a few posts, some updates. I shared the links with close family – it was a way to keep everyone up to speed on what was happening in our lives. But in October 2008, my blog took on new significance. We were at the beginning of what eventually turned out to be just shy of a twelve-month hospital stay. This was the one where Daisy was found to have complete intestinal failure and needed to start on TPN.

I found myself writing furiously during the long hours spent at Daisy's bedside, pouring out my feelings, sharing my thoughts, giving updates on what was happening. The blog became my friend. I barely saw Andy as he tried to keep things going at home. Writing helped me process what was going on, and it also ensured that I directed the narrative to the outside world. If it wasn't on my blog, it wasn't happening.

I began to share my frustrations about the system we found ourselves in, in order to educate those in the 'outside world' – our fight for homecare support, the impact on the family, my worries about Daisy.

It was also a record of our lives, an account of what was happening that our children could look back on in years to come as they reflected on their childhood experience and what had happened. There were very few pictures, just a lot of words.

As my blog posts began to be shared, I was very aware that some of these new readers were not just strangers or other parents; they also included some of the nurses, doctors and professionals who were part of our lives.

It was a tricky balance. I was increasingly aware that I was sharing our family story, and I tried to minimise details about my other children. I tried to be upbeat about Daisy – I wanted blog readers to know her as a little girl with choices and opinions, deserving of a quality of life, but I was also aware that I was doing this on her behalf, telling the world about her when she was not in a position to give me permission or express an opinion on whether she wanted me to do that.

I was not alone. Many parents caring for children with complex needs keep diaries, or some form of blog or record. I recently spoke to a doctor who was doing some research among families using children's hospice services. She had noticed how so many of her interviewees keep online accounts of their lives.

'But you can see why, can't you?' I told her. 'It's just all so surreal. We need to record it so that we can look back and understand what actually happened, and sometimes we just need to reach out and tell other people about what's happening.'

Inevitably, I began to share my blog posts on my social media pages – first Facebook, then increasingly on Twitter and Instagram; I found myself using these channels more and more. But I was still determined to carefully curate what messages I was conveying to the outside world about what was going on in our lives. My other children were now active on social media; I wanted them to feel positive about our lives, not burdened by the experience.

Over the years, I had become very conscious that I needed the health professionals on my side. The words of a mother I met in the neonatal unit had never left me: 'We need them, they don't need us.' It's an utterly wrong approach, but I wanted our professionals to want to work with us, to be pleased when they saw Daisy's name on the outpatients list, to want to go the extra mile for us, not treat me as 'that mother'. I would never name doctors or nurses on social media posts – as far as I'm concerned, that's simply wrong and unethical – but there were times when I would rant about a situation that had occurred – a surgery cancelled at the last minute, missing notes. I didn't want to personally attack individuals; it was the system that frustrated me, and I needed the world to know how that impacted Daisy's life.

Social media is a lifeline for parents caring for children with complex medical needs; it keeps us connected both with the outside world and with other people going through the same experience. There's an immediacy about posting on social media that is very appealing to parents. It can feel less intimidating to ask a question in a parents' forum than in an outpatient appointment or during a ward round. Going online feels like a safe space.

What's important to the parent may be not at the top of the clinician's list of questions to be answered during a meeting. Which says as much about how we feel about the parent/doctor interaction as it does about how parent carers use social media and online forums.

I learned a lot through chatting to other parents online – recommendations for stoma bags that didn't constantly fall off, information about different respite services that were available in my area that our own social worker didn't know about. There was always emotional support, someone who understood, but I still remained careful about how much detail I shared about Daisy and our family.

I was conscious of ensuring that there was a boundary between what I shared online and the minutiae of what was happening at home. I could see how some parents caring for complex children were sharing often quite intimate details of their child's journey. This 'sharenting' presents a narrative over which the child has no control. It's a 'unique clash between a parent's right to make choices for their child and a paediatric patient's right to privacy'.[1]

Putting the child's disability at the centre of the family narrative online makes it the chosen identity for all family members, whether they like it or not. We soon learned to avoid the groups where our circumstance was seen as 'inspiration porn'. I didn't want Daisy to be a warrior or a princess; she was a little girl first and foremost, one of four children. We were an ordinary family who had been thrown into extraordinary circumstances.

---

1   Burn, E. (2021) '#warriors: Sick children, social media and the right to an open future.' *Journal of Medical Ethics* 48, 78. http://dx.doi.org/10.1136/medethics-2020-107042

Parents caring for medically complex children *need* social media; it provides both emotional support and information, and it helps alleviate the loneliness and fear. Time and time again, it was the information and advice that I received from fellow parents that was the most helpful.

Parents have told me that being able to share their experiences by blogging or sharing on social media helps them make sense of their experience. It helps them feel less lonely but, most importantly, it gives them a voice when they feel they are not heard.

Would they be less likely to share if they felt listened to?

I followed an interesting Twitter thread recently where a parent shared that they had found references to their social media account in their child's medical notes and had been told it would be unwise to make comments about their child's care online. This post was followed by a whole slew of responses and anecdotes from parents to the same effect, concerns that 'problem parent' accounts are monitored.

It's a tricky one. Parents need social media – it fulfils a need for support and information about how to care and advocate for their child – but there's a thin line between peer-to-peer support and unqualified advice. Anti-vaxxer disinformation spreads like wildfire on parenting forums, spreading fear and fuelling dissent. Social media platforms have wised up to this and many have systems to manage vaccine misinformation, taking it down quickly and linking to verified sources in return. Social media is uncensored and unmonitored, however, when it comes to the information, advice and images that parents share among special needs and medical communities.

And then there's the next level, where opinions are shared online about hospitals and teams. I remember one very lovely nurse sitting in tears as she read a negative blog about the care a child had received recently on her ward. That episode really hit home. We are all just human beings. The nurse was caught up in a broken system, trying to do her best for the patients, but, unfortunately, she had no right of response, whereas the blog was shared widely with other parents commenting and agreeing with the post.

Social media is part of our everyday life and culture, and it holds an even stronger significance for parents caring for children with medical complexity. It's not an exaggeration to say that it's a lifeline. The world we have entered is so surreal at times that reaching out for support from other parents brings comfort and reassurance. But reaching out to the wider world brings up a whole ethical issue about how much parents should be sharing about their child and the reasons they are even drawn to doing so in the first place.

There is an argument that sharing on social media helps show the reality of our world, and it also helps the wider world face up to the very real fact that sometimes children die or are dependent on machines to live, that sometimes they cannot be cured, that medical science cannot help them. But is this morally and ethically in the child's best interests?

Parents are the primary protectors of their children and should act to protect their child's best interests, especially 'Generation Tagged',[2] the most watched-over generation in memory. Recent, very high-profile cases, have shown how social media can snowball, and the line between a child's right to privacy, enshrined in Article 16 of the UN Convention on the Rights of the Child, is pitted against their parent's right to freedom of expression, guaranteed in Article 13 of the same document.

Breakdowns in communication and trust between parents and the professionals treating their child can spill out on to social media, uniting followers around a hashtag and driving disputes and disagreements outside the hospital walls and into the public domain for all to comment on. The most obvious, high-profile case is that of a baby called Charlie Gard.

Although seemingly normal at birth, Charlie was subsequently diagnosed with an incurable, degenerative mitochondrial disease. The family had barely spent any time home together before he began to show signs of deterioration; at only a few months old, he

---

2   Nottingham, E. (2018) 'Call for greater transparency for Generation Tagged.' The Transparency Project. www.transparencyproject.org.uk/call-for-greater-transparency-for-generation-tagged

was a patient on the paediatric intensive care ward at Great Ormond Street Hospital, and doctors were having conversations with the family about withdrawing life support.

Charlie's parents launched an online fundraising campaign to raise money to take their son to the USA for experimental treatment. They wanted to explore every option for their son and believed that the treatment, although untested on a child with his particular condition at that time, would give them a chance to bring their son home again.

Using the social media hashtags #CharliesArmy and #SaveCharlie, they began a campaign to support their crowdfunding efforts. Charlie's parents shared pictures of their little boy, attached to a ventilator on the intensive care ward, as well as pictures of how he looked before his condition became known and he began to lose function.

I watched on the sidelines as the campaign snowballed. I have seen many crowdfunding campaigns over the years, but this one seemed to follow a trajectory that was unprecedented. Money poured in and the drama played out on Twitter. It seemed everyone had an opinion about this child and his treatment, what the doctors should and should not do, and who was right and wrong.

Crowds gathered outside Great Ormond Street Hospital to protest about Charlie's care, police were called in to investigate death threats to hospital staff,[3] and the hospital was subject to a tirade of online abuse. A student nurse who had been one of Daisy's carers told me that she was working a night shift on one ward and answered a call to the nurses station to be greeted by the scream 'Murderer!'

The press picked up on the campaign, the hashtags trended daily, and then the awareness skyrocketed as both the Pope and President Trump tweeted their support for Charlie's parents.

I was struck with so many mixed emotions and feelings. I had

---

3   Connett, D. (2017) 'Great Ormond Street staff "get death threats" over Charlie Gard.' *The Guardian*, 22 July. www.theguardian.com/uk-news/2017/jul/22/great-ormond-street-staff-receive-death-threats-over-charlie-gard

walked a similar path but made different decisions. I was even momentarily questioning my own decision: should I have tried harder for Daisy? I was concerned about the comments from 'armchair medics' online – no one knew the precise details of Charlie's condition apart from his own medical team and his parents. While the parents and Charlie's Army were able to comment on Twitter and in the press, the hospital could only issue statements, bound as they were by the need to protect the privacy of their patient, Charlie.

As I watched the drama play out, I wondered if the family felt at any stage that the campaign had snowballed to the extent that others were using it for their own agenda.

In the aftermath, Rajana Das, a sociologist at the University of Surrey blogged about the impact of the campaign and the role of 'Charlie's Army':

> By employing some classic markers of populism, the 'army' has demonstrated a kind of 'networked populism' which has co-opted evidence-based debate into the territory of heightened, emotive responses between and across strangers. These have ranged from genuine anguish and expressions of sorrow, to the use of terminology from the Third Reich to characterise doctors, lawyers and clinicians, and to displaying overwhelming emotions of feeling at one with and attached to the real-time tweeting of court hearings, almost as though these were televisual narratives unfolding.[4]

Building on this, Das also analysed the 'twitterstorm' that ensued during the Charlie Gard case. She found that many of the tweets around the #CharliesArmy hashtag emanated from US-based accounts, many of whom identified as having right-wing positions.

Her analysis found that the tweets in support of the campaign showed:

---

4   Das, R. (2017) 'Key lessons from the role of the media in the Charlie Gard case.' Department of Sociology, University of Surrey, blog post, 8 August. https://blogs.surrey.ac.uk/sociology/2017/08/08/key-lessons-from-the-role-of-the-media-in-the-charlie-gard-case

a heavy and sustained use of single words, repeatedly, all of which conjure up an image of violence and devastation inflicted on a vulnerable individual by an unknowable, strange, powerful hospital. The top words in this category are – devastated, heart-breaking, cruel, death panel, loss, tragic and threaten.[5]

The Charlie Gard case changed things. There had been other high-profile awareness and fundraising campaigns initiated by families, but this was on another level and created a rhetoric of conflict between institutions (the hospital) and the family that seemed to be unprecedented. The hospital was portrayed as holding Charlie hostage, of signing his death warrant, of undermining parental rights.

And the prevailing tone among the parent community was 'if you're not with us, you're against us'. I wanted to remain impartial; I did not want to pass judgement on a situation that I had no right to pass judgement on. The only people who had the full facts on the case were the people in the room with Charlie. Yet those who disagreed with the family were accused of being trolls.

But thousands of online supporters agreed with the family's actions. Many were well-meaning, but many had their own agenda to push: religious, pro-life, anti-socialised healthcare. At times, I wondered what Charlie's parents thought of it all. Their lives on public view, their dying child on public view and the whole world, from President Trump to the Pope, it appeared, had an opinion on what they should and should not do.

I approached Charlie's mum, Connie, and asked her if she would be prepared to be interviewed for this book and give her account; sadly, she declined. I wanted to learn more about Charlie's story and her experiences and feelings. I stumbled across an interview she had given for a podcast series. It threw up more questions and also a moment of chilling realisation. She was explaining to the

5   Das, R. (2017) 'The Charlie Gard twitterstorm: A violent and negative impact (new research).' LSE blog post, 4 August. https://blogs.lse.ac.uk/polis/2017/08/04/the-charlie-gard-twitterstorm-a-violent-and-negative-impact-new-research

interviewer how, in hindsight, she had PTSD from her experience caring for her son.

As I listened, I realised in a moment of chilling realisation that she might even have been describing the moment when Daisy had a cardiac arrest, only hours before her death:

> I was in the family room one day, which was right next to intensive care, and the emergency alarm went off, and you know, it's this deafening sound and you think, oh my God, is that my baby? ... It's a haunting sound, and every parent's the same, you see the look on their faces if they're in the room with you...whose child is that? You run down the corridor...it wasn't Charlie and you think, Thank God, then you realise that's someone else's child...you feel guilty that it's not your child but you don't want it to be anyone's child.[6]

Connie did what she needed to do for her son. Ass she said in the podcast, if she could go back, knowing what she knows now, she would have approached things differently. I did what I needed to do for my daughter. We both had very different ways of managing the situation we found ourselves in, and for very different reasons. There are no right or wrong decisions – just awful, difficult, heart-rending decisions that stay with you for the rest of your life.

The Charlie Gard case was a game-changer in many ways; it highlighted the extremes some parents are willing to go to in order to ensure no stone is unturned in the quest for a treatment for their child, but it also showed the power of social media in helping raise both funds to pay for potential treatments and awareness of the case.

The narrative became combative rather than collaborative, a battle to be won with the child a #Warrior and #Fighter. It felt as though this became a turning point in how parents, and the wider public, viewed the professionals treating children with complex needs – portrayed in the media as unfeeling and uncaring faceless

---

6   Coulson, A. (n.d.) 'Crisis what crisis?' Interview with Connie Yates. https://thecharliegardfoundation.org/crisis-what-crisis

institutions, they had no voice to counter this narrative apart from official channels.

Yet these were very real human beings who were caught up in this whole situation, who could not speak out or voice an opinion, who were trying to do their best and care for a very sick child while the media storm raged outside.

A year after Daisy died, I met up with a couple of the nurses who had been on the intensive care ward and cared for her the day she died. I asked them about the Charlie Gard case. They were clearly shaken and traumatised by the whole experience and refused to be drawn into any discussion – they had probably been told they were not allowed to – but one of them commented that it was really obvious how behaviours had changed among some parents since that time:

'They say things like "I know my rights", and they refuse to be discharged from the intensive care unit even though their child doesn't need that level of support,' she told me.

In 2018, another similar case began to unfold, this time in Liverpool's Alder Hey Children's Hospital. Again, a social media 'Army' was assembled to support little Alfie Evans who had been diagnosed with another very rare mitochondrial disease. This time, there was no hope of a potentially untried and untested treatment at stake. The hospital said scans showed 'catastrophic degradation of his brain tissue' and that further treatment was not only 'futile' but also 'unkind and inhumane'.[7] Alfie's parents wanted to take him to a hospital in Italy for treatment that would not improve his condition but simply prolong his life for an unspecified time.

I watched again as the hashtag #AlfiesArmy trended on Twitter and Alfie's parents, barely older than my older son, posted picture after picture of their son online.

The final days of Alfie's life were played out on social media, with hospital statements contrasting with a stream of video and picture updates online. Crowds were gathered outside the hospital,

7   www.judiciary.uk/wp-content/uploads/2018/02/alder-hey-v-evans.pdf

security was increased, staff were told to cover their uniforms when leaving the building, parents were escorted to their child's bedside when visiting wards...

I watched as Alfie's distraught father live-streamed video of his son, still breathing despite being extubated but clearly (to those who know how to recognise the signs) in his final stages of life. It begs the question, 'Should social media channels have a role to play to protect the privacy of dying children, ensuring that their final, deeply intimate moments are not shared around the world?'

There have been more high-profile cases, pitting parents against hospitals online. Hospitals have developed policies to manage such high-profile cases, to protect the anonymity of staff and patients. Not all of them trend so publicly online but one fundamental question remains.

What drives parents to use social media to air their grievances so publicly? How did relationships and trust break down so badly to drive it to that point?

There's one common theme that surfaces with every parent I have spoken to: they just want their voices to be heard.

CHAPTER 16

No Stone Unturned

T HANKS TO THE HUMAN GENOME PROJECT'S[1] ground-breaking work, we were among the first in the world to learn that
Daisy's condition was caused by a mutation on the HRAS gene.
That confirmation opened up a whole world of potential to understand her condition. The fact that the HRAS gene is an oncogene[2]
was significant in ensuring that we screened her regularly for cancer.
Knowing more about how Costello syndrome occurred helped the
doctors and geneticists studying this very rare disease. The mapping
of the human genome heralded a revolution in medicine, opening
up a whole world of potential treatments and therapies for patients
diagnosed with genetic diseases.

The constantly evolving world of medical devices and technology has also meant that children who could once only be cared for
in a hospital environment or by specialist nurses can now be cared
for at home by their parents. Clever gadgets and medical tech meant
that I could change Daisy's gastrostomy and jejunostomy tubes at
home, check her blood sugar and administer growth-hormone
injections, all thanks to nifty, almost foolproof, medical devices.
The ability to use mobile TPN pumps with automatic programmes
literally changed our lives. No longer did we have to rely on big blue
IVAC pumps clamped to IV poles that tested my muscle strength;

---

1   www.genome.gov/human-genome-project
2   A gene associated with cancer.

instead, portable pumps meant that Daisy could get out and about. Crucial when she became 24/7 TPN dependent.

We took Daisy to the USA when she was very little, in the days before TPN. We wanted to attend the bi-annual gathering of the Costello Syndrome Family Support Network. We knew that the scientists leading the work into potential treatments for this rare condition would be in attendance. We hoped that they might give us some insights, the chance to participate in a trial, an opportunity for a new treatment.

Getting to the US required a lot of effort. We applied for grants, we saved, we fundraised, and assembling everything we needed, together with all the relevant medical documentation, was a military operation.

But we did it, and we flew to the West Coast of the USA, just so that the doctors who were at the forefront of research into Daisy's rare condition could meet her and we could see if there were any ideas for how we could help her live the best quality of life.

We learned that there was lots of research happening, all in very early stages, and any clinical trials were still a long way off. We were given some useful information on screening protocols to look for potential cancer and heart problems, and copies of papers that would help Daisy's endocrinologist make decisions about the pros and cons of treating her unstable blood sugars with growth-hormone injections. No potential treatments or miracle cures, but still worth every bit of effort to ensure that we left no stone unturned in our quest to maximise Daisy's quality of life, to make the most of our finite time with her.

On reflection, I doubt if Andy and I would have subjected Daisy to any untried and untested treatments, no matter how much we wanted to have her around in our lives for as long as possible. I didn't want her to be the guinea pig; I needed to be confident that whatever treatment or therapy we tried would be beneficial for her and not cause her any further harm.

What if we had been given the option to try a completely new and untested treatment for her? There's lots of work underway to find treatments that will dampen down the worst effects of Costello syndrome. If Daisy had been offered the opportunity to be one of the first to test this treatment, my instinct is that I would have said no until we knew whether there was any more evidence. But who knows? And who am I to judge other parents who choose differently?

Charlie Gard's parents stated that they wanted him to have a three-month trial of an experimental nucleoside therapy treatment which had been tested on mice. A human trial of children with a slightly different mutation to Charlie had shown some minor improvements. There was no firm evidence that the therapy repaired the damage caused to the brain in the rare disease it targeted or that it would work on the specific mutation found in Charlie's case, but it was considered by the team researching the therapy in the US to be relatively risk-free.[3]

However, electrical tracings of Charlie's brain (EEG) found that his condition had deteriorated to a point that his doctors believed that treatment would be 'futile and only prolong Charlie's suffering'.[4]

The outcome was a disagreement between the parents and clinicians about what was in Charlie's best interests and the launch of a fundraising campaign by Charlie's parents to take him to the US for treatment. That was their bid to leave no stone unturned in pursuing treatment for their son.

The wonderful work unravelling the human genome and the revolution it's triggered in medicine has created complex ethical dilemmas for medical professionals to consider. Increasingly, they face the question, 'Just because we can, does it mean we should?'

As with all ethical dilemmas, there are no easy solutions, and there may not be a single right answer. Every person is different. What was right for Daisy would not be right for another family.

3   Kegel, M. (2017) 'Nucleoside therapy explained: Why doctors hesitate to treat Charlie Gard.' Mitochondrial Disease News, 19 July. https://mitochondrialdiseasenews.com/2017/07/19/nucleoside-therapy-explained-why-doctors-debate-treating-charlie-gard

4   Wilkinson, D. and Savulescu, J. (2018) 'The Charlie Gard case.' In Ethics, Conflict and Medical Treatment for Children: From Disagreement to Dissensus. Elsevier Health Sciences.

In facing seemingly impossible decisions, clinicians need to consider the four pillars of medical ethics:

- **Respect for autonomy** – helping patients (or, in the case of children, the person who speaks for them) to make reasoned and informed choices about their care and treatment.

- **Non-maleficence** – the fundamental basis of medicine, 'first do no harm'; any harm should not be disproportionate to the benefits of the treatment being proposed.

- **Beneficence** – medical professionals should always act in a way which benefits the patient. It's about 'doing good' for the patient but also considering what's acceptable for them.

- **Justice** – here, the consideration is whether the proposed treatment is compatible with the law and the patient's rights, and if it's fair and balanced. Within the NHS system in the UK, this principle is also applied to ensure no one is unfairly disadvantaged when it comes to access to healthcare.

Medical professionals face increasingly complex and difficult dilemmas as scientific progress provides more options and possibilities for treatments and care. In turn, the discipline of clinical ethics is growing rapidly as medical professionals seek advice and support in making seemingly impossible decisions for their patients.

The question at the heart of such ethically challenging decisions will always be 'What constitutes an acceptable quality of life?'

And how do we measure that?

Charlie's family were prepared to take him overseas for an untried treatment in order to gain even a minimal improvement and to extend his life. Conversely, when Andy and I discussed how far we were prepared to go with treatments in order to extend Daisy's life, we both agreed that should her airway fail to the point that she would need a tracheostomy in order to breathe, this was a step we were not prepared to take for her.

We were fortunate to have time to consider these issues before any crisis hit. We had time with Daisy, her decline was long and slow, and we had the benefit of a very early referral to palliative care services before Daisy was at end of life. This gave us an opportunity to think about what we felt was important for Daisy, what she would want us to do, what, for us, constituted an acceptable quality of life, how far we were prepared to go with treatment and what that would enable.

Nikki, Lennon's mum, shared with me how she and her partner, Ian, had similar conversations about how far they would go in his treatment – at what point would they say 'enough is enough'.

'For us, it was TPN,' she told me. 'Lennon now had an ileostomy. We were struggling with that – his learning disability coupled with his mobility meant that managing that alone was hard enough. We just knew that TPN would have been a nightmare to manage safely with him; it would put him at greater risk. We knew it was not an option that would ultimately enhance his quality of life.'

Those conversations came about not with a palliative doctor or team, however, but with a nurse specialist who had become the family's trusted professional. She knew Nikki and Ian well enough to ask the question 'How far are you prepared to go in treating Lennon?' The couple trusted her; they knew that she understood what life was like caring for their son 24/7, and they knew that these were open and honest conversations that they could have with her, borne out of a mutual understanding of what was important in achieving a good quality of life for Lennon.

When her son Matthias was diagnosed with an extremely rare, fast-growing prostatic tumour, Rosie was told that proton beam therapy treatment would give him the best chance of a cure. I was surprised when she told me that the NHS funded her son's treatment at a specialist centre in the USA as there was no suitable proton beam therapy centre in the UK at the time.

The financial support only covered the costs for Matthias and one parent, so the family fundraised to ensure that they could all be together during his time in treatment.

Ultimately, the treatment was unsuccessful. Despite this, Rosie has the happiest memories of that time: 'It was the best three months of our lives because we were together as a family. And we did jolly things when we were in Florida. We did the whole tourist thing, and we made wonderful memories together,' she told me.

As far as Rosie is concerned, they tried. There was hope that this would be the cure that would bring their beloved son back and give him back his childhood. It didn't, but she doesn't regret a single moment of trying.

I hadn't actually realised that proton beam therapy treatment was available and funded by the NHS in a non-UK hospital until I began to research this book.

The idea of using proton beams in a medical context was first developed in 1946, and the first hospital-based proton beam therapy treatment centre opened in California in 1991. Proton beam therapy is a more targeted form of radiotherapy, which has the potential to cause fewer or milder side effects than traditional radiotherapy. It's no wonder parents are prepared to fight for this treatment for their child. Wouldn't you if you had a sick child and turned to Google to find out what else was available?

It's still a relatively new treatment, and, according to NHS England:

> Proton beam therapy is only suitable for certain types of cancer, such as highly complex brain, head and neck cancers and sarcomas as it does not lead to better outcomes for many cancer cases than using high energy x-rays, which is still considered the most appropriate and effective treatment for the majority of cancers.[5]

There are now two centres in the UK offering the treatment, but the NHS continues to fund some patients who fulfil a strict set of criteria to access treatment abroad.

What if your child doesn't fulfil the funding criteria? What if their oncologist recommended 'traditional' radiotherapy over

---

5   NHS (n.d.) 'Proton beam therapy.' www.england.nhs.uk/commissioning/spec-services/highly-spec-services/pbt

targeted proton beam therapy? How would you feel knowing that a potential treatment exists that could offer less harmful long-term side effects for your child? You might consider going to great lengths to try to get that treatment.

That's what happened in two high-profile cases.

In 2012, Sally Roberts found herself in the headlines. She had gone into hiding with her son, Neon. The police were hunting for her as she was accused of preventing Neon's treatment for a malignant brain tumour.

Neon's doctors had recommended a course of radiotherapy and chemotherapy following surgery to remove the tumour, but Sally had disagreed with this plan, despite it being the 'gold standard' of the time. Writing in her blog, she says that she had explored less invasive, more targeted treatment options for her son and had begun fundraising in order to take Neon to the USA in order to undergo proton beam therapy.[6] At the time, the press vilified Sally for her interest in exploring alternative therapy options instead of agreeing to radiotherapy.

Sally was prepared to go on the run with her son because she was concerned that the treatment being proposed would affect his future quality of life. 'I wanted the best treatment for my son and I didn't think at that time radiation was necessary because he was already cancer-free,' she told *The Guardian*, a year later.[7] By this point, Neon had been made a ward of court and the recommended radiotherapy treatment course had been completed.

It's interesting looking back at some of the press reports and coverage at the time. In an interview with the *Daily Mail*, Sally mentions a conversation with her son's oncologist:

We were talking about lots of things to do with Neon's treatment. The doctor said he would need radiotherapy across all his brain.

6   Roberts, S.J. (2020) *The Treatment: 'First Do No Harm'*. Matador.
7   Davies, C. (2012) 'Neon Roberts's mother refused time to seek alternative tumour treatments.' *The Guardian*, 20 December. www.theguardian.com/society/2012/dec/20/neon-roberts-mother-time-tumour

When I questioned why they couldn't target only the area where the tumour was, he replied: 'You have to fry the whole brain.' He immediately said: 'Oh, I shouldn't have put it like that.' But I was horrified.[8]

Was that throwaway comment the tipping point – did it set off the train of events that followed? That led Sally to go on the run? For Neon to be made a ward of court?

Parents hang on to every word their children's doctors tell them, so a poorly judged comment can have huge ramifications.

Neon's story has familiar echoes in another high-profile case a few years later. Ashya King was another little boy with a brain tumour whose family took him out of hospital, and out of the country, in order to pursue their aim of treating him with proton beam therapy rather than conventional radiotherapy. High-profile media coverage followed, and, at one point, Ashya's parents found themselves imprisoned after an international police hunt tracked them to their holiday home in Spain.

Ashya's doctors insist they took a clinical and not a financial decision that proton beam therapy would not be better for him than conventional radiotherapy.[9] His parents disagreed. They had done their own research online and were prepared to sell their holiday home in order to fund the treatment, which they believed would be better for their son. In their view, the treatment proposed by Ashya's clinical team would 'turn him into a vegetable'. The hospital treating Ashya referred his case to a specialist panel which considered the merits and benefits of proton beam therapy treatment on a case-by-case basis. The expert panel confirmed the hospital's opinion that Ashya was not a suitable candidate.

8   Clarke, N. and Bentley, P. (2012) '"Am I ever going to see you again Mummy?" What Neon, 7, cried as he was snatched by social workers from mother who took him on the run to block life-saving cancer treatment.' *Daily Mail*, 7 December. www.dailymail.co.uk/news/article-2244853/Sally-Roberts-Am-I-going-Mummy-What-Neon-7-cried-snatched-social-workers.html

9   Smith, J. (2014) 'Ashya King: This story isn't quite what it seems.' *Independent*, 9 September. www.independent.co.uk/voices/comment/ashya-king-story-isn-t-quite-what-it-seems-9716486.html

His parent's actions eventually brought Ashya's case into the media spotlight. They took his case to court, where it was ruled that the little boy could have proton beam therapy treatment, to be funded by the NHS. This was despite his clinical team's continuing insistence that the treatment would have the same side effects as conventional radiotherapy.

Ashya was eventually treated at a clinic in Prague. He's alive today but continues to live with the side effects of his cancer and treatment.

His case exposed many issues. It was hugely emotive and dominated the news headlines. Hospital staff were subjected to abuse[10] in a chilling precursor of the tirade of hatred and trolling that fell out of the Charlie Gard and Alfie Evans cases which followed a few years later.

Dr Peter Wilson, one of the doctors caring for Ashya at the time, later commented in a BBC documentary, *Ashya: The Untold Story*:

> It does put clinicians in an impossible position because we now have to try to explain to families why one child...is getting a form of treatment, why they can't and they've got the same tumour... And that's deeply unfair when the NHS is supposed to be about equal healthcare for all.[11]

Following the Ashya King case, a safeguarding review was conducted to look at what had happened and lessons that could be learned. The review concluded that, in general, agencies acted appropriately and that, in the context in which professionals were working, there was little that could have been done differently. But they also highlighted the breakdown in communication with Ashya's parents and how the actions of the professionals had contributed to this.

One factor that is relevant was a delay in obtaining a second

10 Press Association (2015) 'Hospital in Ashya King case reveals "outpouring of hatred" directed at staff.' *The Guardian*, 10 April. www.theguardian.com/uk-news/2015/apr/10/hospital-in-ashya-king-case-reveals-outpouring-of-hatred-directed-at-staff

11 www.bbc.co.uk/programmes/b05qyjl9

opinion for the parents. Whilst the doctors' view that this was not needed immediately was accurate in terms of the child's clinical needs, this failed to take account of the indirect message that was given to the parents, which was that their wishes and rights were overruled by the professionals.[12]

Communication again...listening to the family's concerns. It might not have affected the outcome, but as the report states:

The review provides an opportunity for professionals to reflect on the unintended consequences of decisions including the need for professionals to examine their actions from the point of view of the parent and child. Reassurance of patients and parents is a vital element of care and sometimes it is necessary to spend time enabling parents to get a second opinion even if it will not change the clinical outcome, in order that parents can feel that they have explored all possible avenues.

Exploring every possible avenue...that resonated with me. I knew deep down that Daisy would not be a candidate for transplant surgery to replace her diseased bowel, liver and stomach. My instinct told me that it would likely do more harm than good and certainly would not solve all of her issues. But I still needed to know that the professionals were listening to me when I asked about transplant, rather than just dismissing my requests for a transplant review and assessment. As it was, just a simple presentation of her case to the transplant team yielded the answers I needed. Daisy's team knew she would not be a candidate, but at least I felt I'd explored every possible avenue, that my concerns were being heard.

There was another important element to the Ashya King case. The family were devout followers of the Jehovah's Witness religion. Early press coverage about the case focused on this, spotlighting the fact that people who practise that religion are forbidden from

---

12 Portsmouth Safeguarding Board (2015) Executive Summary of the lessons learned from a review of inter-agency working with a child in acute care. www.portsmouthscb.org.uk/wp-content/uploads/EXECUTIVE-SUMMARY-Final-5-9-15.pdf

receiving blood transfusions. It was suggested the parents might have escaped hospital to keep their son from receiving blood transfusions, necessary in radiotherapy and chemotherapy treatments.[13]

The narrative shifted when it became clear that the driver behind the parents' actions in taking their son from hospital was to ensure that he received proton beam therapy treatment.

While there were no faith reasons behind the actions of Ashya's parents, religious tenets and beliefs can sometimes be a central element in conflicts and disagreements around a child's care.

How do these impact the decisions that parents and clinicians face in how far to go in treating a child? And where can each party turn for support and guidance?

13 Sapiña, L., Ligero, S. and Dominguez, M. (2018) 'Protons for Jehovah's Witnesses? How press coverage of Ashya King's case brought proton beam therapy to the public sphere.' *Estudios sobre el Mensaje Periodístico*. http://dx.doi.org/10.5209/ESMP.62246

CHAPTER 17

A Question of Faith

W HEN ANDY WAS DIAGNOSED WITH CANCER, he made it very clear that he did not want anyone to pray for him or offer him hopes of a cure rooted in some strange diet or ceremony or visit to a holy shrine. He was very much a confirmed atheist who put his faith in science and in the skills of the team caring for him.

I am probably not as fierce in my opposition to religion as my late husband. It comes from my anthropology training and my international education. I've always tried to see the world through other people's eyes and understand the cultural and social influences that drive their actions. I know people of all faiths and none, and many of them were people who cared for Daisy. I respected them all, I thanked them for their prayers, but I'm guided by science, logic and my own moral compass. And then there's always an element of the lapsed Catholic that emerges in times of crisis.

But for some people, faith plays a significant role in the decisions they make on behalf of their child.

That's a difficult path for healthcare professionals to tread. In some cases, there are clear guidelines to help them navigate disagreements in caring for a child where the family's faith plays a major factor in how they should be treated. There are protocols to support clinicians who are caring for patients who are Jehovah's Witnesses, for example. Although not opposed to surgery or medicine, Jehovah's Witnesses decline allogenic blood transfusion for reasons of religious faith. This is a deeply held core value, and any non-consensual transfusion is regarded as a gross physical violation.

When a child from a family that adheres to Jehovah's Witness principles requires a life-saving blood transfusion, then there are legal precedents that can assist clinicians. Children aged 16 or 17 can give legally valid consent for medical treatment, whereas children under this age can give consent if they are deemed to have a sufficient level of competency to understand the issues involved (I discuss Gillick competence in later chapters). Jehovah's Witnesses maintain a network of hospital liaison committees that are available at any time to assist with the management of patients, either at the request of the patient or (with patient consent) on behalf of the treating team.

But what about situations where parents take a religious stance in insisting on continuing life-sustaining treatment for their child, where clinicians feel it is not in their best interests?

In 2021, a case where religious tenets pitted parents against clinicians brought this issue into the headlines.

Alta Fixsler was born prematurely in December 2018 but sadly suffered catastrophic brain injuries at birth. She was resuscitated and ventilated and remained in hospital. The clinicians managing Alta's care told her parents that, in their view, it was unlikely that she would live beyond the age of two. They also believed she was experiencing pain and had no conscious awareness. Tests revealed that most of Alta's brain structure had been lost. She was unable to maintain an open airway and breathe independently, blink her eyes, maintain her core body temperature or hear. They advised her parents that, in their view and based on the tests, there was no chance of recovery.[1]

As devout Hasidic Jews, Alta's parents maintained that their faith was not simply a religion but a way of life. They disagreed with Alta's doctor's opinion that it was in her best interests to remove life-sustaining treatment.

---

1   *Manchester University NHS Foundation Trust v Fixsler & Ors* [2021] EWHC 1426 (Fam), www.judiciary.uk/wp-content/uploads/2022/07/Manchester-University-NHS-Foundation-Trust-v-Fixsler-judgment.pdf

Alta's case went before the Royal Court of Justice in May 2021, once again pitting clinician against parent with a very sick child at the centre.

Confirming their opposition to removal of life-supporting treatment on religious grounds Alta'a parents gave this statement to the court:

> We are practicing Ultra-Orthodox Jews who adhere to what we are instructed to do in line with the Torah and Jewish faith. We are taught that life is sacred and not only must we preserve life, we also cannot be involved in bringing death closer... In our faith, it is strictly forbidden to actively shorten a life. The only circumstances under which this might be permissible is where somebody is in constant suffering and pain, but we do not believe that these circumstances apply to Alta.[2]

The presiding judge focused on the medical evidence that pointed to the fact that Alta was indeed experiencing pain and that her pain would likely worsen and her condition deteriorate, and that it was therefore not in her best interests to maintain artificial ventilation in order to keep her alive. In his decision he took into account 'the fact that continuing life sustaining treatment will confine Alta to being kept alive for the remainder of her life in a hospital room without windows, her life sustained by machines in a world she cannot meaningfully perceive or connect with.'[3] He also felt that complying with her parent's wish to transfer Alta to a hospital in Israel to continue life-sustaining treatment would cause the child unnecessary pain.

The judge considered the religious arguments for sustaining Alta's life support that had been put to the court by her parent's legal team and their Rabbi. While he agreed that the family's Jewish belief system was certainly one element to be taken into account

2   *Manchester University NHS Foundation Trust v Fixsler & Ors* [2021] EWHC 1426 (Fam). www.judiciary.uk/wp-content/uploads/2022/07/Manchester-University-NHS-Foundation-Trust-v-Fixsler-judgment.pdf, paragraph 50.

3   *Manchester University NHS Foundation Trust v Fixsler & Ors* [2021] EWHC 1426 (Fam). www.judiciary.uk/wp-content/uploads/2022/07/Manchester-University-NHS-Foundation-Trust-v-Fixsler-judgment.pdf, paragraph 103.

when considering a best interests decision about Alta, it should not be based on the assumption that *she* would share the same values and beliefs as her family and community.

When a case involving a disagreements between parents and the child's clinicians reaches family court, a guardian is appointed by the Children and Family Court Advisory and Support Service (CAFCASS). The role of the CAFCASS guardian is to represent the rights and interests of the child. They appoint the child's own separate legal representation for the case. The aim here is ensure that the child is seen as independent of their parents, that their views and opinions are considered as best they can, in order to make objective, rather than emotional decisions on their care.

I used to wonder what it would be like to be transported into Daisy's body and feel what it was like to be her. I could only have a subjective, value judgement on Daisy's quality of life, and this would always be guided by the fact that I had a deep emotional connection to her as her mother.

In Alta's case, the judge acknowledged the family's deeply held faith in preserving life but reminded the court that the case was being judged by secular law. In his summing up, he noted that taking into account the family's religious beliefs would constitute a subjective approach which could not drive a best interests decision but, rather, should form an element of that decision.

He added that:

> [T]he sanctity of Alta's life is not, within the context of the secular laws that this court must apply, absolute. It may, on the facts of an individual case, give way to countervailing factors. In short, the presumption in favour of taking all steps to preserve life, whilst strong, is also rebuttable. That this is so recognises that life cannot be, and indeed should not be preserved at all costs.[4]

Following an unsuccessful appeal to the European Court of Human

---

4 *Manchester University NHS Foundation Trust v Fixsler & Ors* [2021] EWHC 1426 (Fam). www.judiciary.uk/wp-content/uploads/2022/07/Manchester-University-NHS-Foundation-Trust-v-Fixsler-judgment.pdf, paragraph 98.

Rights, Alta was moved to a children's hospice where her ventilator was switched off and her breathing tube removed and, with her parents at her side, she died.

There is absolutely no doubt that the guiding principles of their religion were central to Alta's parents' life and their fight to keep her alive. But I wonder if some parents, desperately searching for a way to keep their child alive, are more susceptible to the influence of religion? I remember looking up to the sky when it was clear that Daisy was entering her final hours of life and silently mouthing, 'You can't have her yet.' I don't know who 'you' was – was it the God that I no longer believed in? Was it her deceased father who had died only 13 months previously?

We cling on to hope for a miracle at our most vulnerable. There's a saying that 'there are no atheists in the trenches'.[5]

I was looking through media reports and court papers while researching this book and found myself drawn to the role religious influence played in the Alfie Evans case. The family campaigned to be allowed to remove Alfie from the hospital where he was being treated in Liverpool to the Bambino Gesù Children's Hospital in the Vatican, Rome. The plan was that he would receive a tracheostomy and gastrostomy in order to maintain his life, but the doctors treating him concluded that moving Alfie would cause him pain and distress and that his brain function had deteriorated to the point that he was in a semi-vegetative state with minimal brain function and no chance of improvement, let alone recovery.

Lengthy court battles ensued, and at one point, Alfie's father, Thomas Evans, flew to the Vatican for a 20-minute audience with the Pope, who later tweeted his support for the family. In the latter weeks of the legal action, the family were supported on a pro bono basis by the Christian Legal Centre (CLC). The CLC state that they work with clients 'taking a stand for Jesus'.[6] The organisation

---

5   Quote Investigator (n.d.) 'There are no atheists in foxholes.' https://quoteinvestigator.com/2016/11/02/foxhole

6   Christian Concern (2023) 'Christian Legal Centre.' https://christianconcern.com/about/services/christian-legal-centre

already had a reputation for supporting high-profile cases concerning religious freedoms[7] and provided Alfie's parents, who had no legal representation at the time, with a barrister and the services of a law student called Pavel Stroilov. Stroilov provided Alfie's father with a letter advising him (incorrectly) that it would be legal to remove his son from the hospital where he was being treated, an action which the hospital's legal team blamed for 'causing a highly-charged standoff between Evans, the police and doctors and ignited protests outside'.[8]

In his commentary on the appeal court submission, Lord Justice MacFarlane raised concerns about how vulnerable and desperate parents can find themselves targeted by organisations (by implication the CLC) who have their own agenda:

> It may be that some investigation of whether, in this country, at this time, parents who find themselves in these awful circumstances, and are therefore desperate for help and vulnerable to engaging with people whose interests may not in fact assist the parents' case, needs some wider investigation.[9]

In 2022, the CLC was back in court in 2022 supporting the family of Archie Battersbee,[10] a young boy who had suffered a catastrophic brain injury at home. His clinical team had recommended that it was in Archie's best interests that life-sustaining treatment was withdrawn as there was no hope of recovery. The case dominated the media as the family appealed against court decisions. Archie

7   Doward, J. and Wheeler, S. (2011) 'Christian Legal Centre fights more than 50 religious discrimination cases.' *The Observer*, 1 May. www.theguardian.com/world/2011/may/01/christianity-rights-colin-atkinson

8   Halliday, J. (2018) 'Legal watchdog may investigate Christian group over Alfie Evans case.' *The Guardian*, 2 May. www.theguardian.com/law/2018/may/02/legal-watchdog-may-investigate-christian-group-over-alfie-evans-case

9   *Mr Thomas Evans v Alder Hey Children's NHS Foundation Trust* [2018] EWCA Civ 984. www.judiciary.uk/wp-content/uploads/2018/05/evans-v-alder-hey-appeal-judgment.pdf

10 Christian Concern (2022) 'Archie Battersbee: Why we supported his family's legal battle.' https://christianconcern.com/comment/archie-battersbee-he-deserves-a-fighting-chance

died in August 2022 after weeks of legal arguments and appeals which played out across the media. Reflecting on the case, commentators believe that the CLC may not have given the family a fair assessment of their chances, giving them false hope.[11]

I can understand how parents can feel be vulnerable in these situations, reaching out for answers, for someone to help them. A few weeks before Daisy died, it was becoming abundantly clear that her quality of life was fading, she was able to do less and less. I remember feeling troubled that while she was not at end of life, I was in some way 'playing God' by putting up the TPN and administering the drugs that were keeping her alive. I felt I had no one to talk to about these feelings; I didn't want to burden family members, and I knew the doctors and nurses caring for Daisy would only be able to give me a clinical opinion; they couldn't tell me what I could or should do – whether I was right or wrong in having these thoughts.

Although I enjoyed escaping to the peace and quiet of the chapel in Great Ormond Street Hospital while Daisy was a patient, I rarely had any contact with the chaplaincy team there. I just assumed they were there for people who had a devout faith and were looking for spiritual support.

That changed after Daisy died. When she was at end of life, my other three children arrived at the hospital as I needed them to say their goodbyes to their sister. I gave them the choice of whether to be with Daisy when we removed her breathing tube or to sit in a separate room. Theo, my elder son, stayed with me while Xanthe and Jules opted not to be there. I needed to be with my daughter as she took her final breaths. A few days later, I discovered that Romana, a Muslim chaplain who was on duty for the chaplaincy team that day, had sat with my other children as they waited to be told their sister had died. I was so grateful that they were not alone at that time and that there was another person in the room with

---

11 Woolley, S. (2022) 'Religious fundamentalist lawyers "preyed on" Archie Battersbee's family.' openDemocracy. www.opendemocracy.net/en/archie-battersbee-christian-legal-centre-preying-whitewash

them. Not talking but just being there when I couldn't. Being a human being.

I wanted to understand how chaplains support parents when there are disagreements with the medical team on their child's treatment. How do they support families where faith principles guide their decisions, even when they are at odds with the clinicians?

I contacted Romana to find out more about her work in the hospital.

'In the Muslim faith,' she told me, 'the guidance is clear: if two doctors are agreed that artificially extending life with mechanical support will prolong a person's suffering, then that support should be removed in order to give the patient dignity and respect in death.'

Just as Islam gives clear guidance on how to support a child when they come into the world, there is guidance on how to support them in death. 'It's about dignity and respect,' she explained. 'And in prolonging their suffering, you are harming them and not treating them in the way that our laws say a dying person should be treated.'

She told me, 'When I sit with families I can see their pain, and they are so concerned about doing the right thing that they can lose sight of their child in the middle of it all.' Doing the right thing can mean following their faith or it can be responding to the influence of others – other family members, people outside their world. There are so many voices advising them, as Romana told me, that it's as though they become paralysed in knowing what to do for their child.

So Romana will often find herself supporting a family who are wrestling with the awful news that the doctors have told them that there is nothing more that can be done for their child. In the majority of cases where she becomes involved, the family are new to this world of complex needs and they are looking for someone to help make sense of it all. It is very much an advocacy role, helping the family find their voice, carrying their burden alongside them and discussing the faith implications. It's clear that in their work, Romana and her colleagues in the hospital chaplaincy team have a great impact, helping families at the worst time in their lives. They speak for them but also have the trust of the clinicians and act as a bridge between the two, sharing the burden, understanding the drivers of faith.

'Sometimes,' Romana told me, 'there's something holding the family back that they just can't articulate to the clinicians, but through spending time with them, it comes out and we can find a way through it.'

She told me a beautiful story to illustrate this that I just have to share; it really moved me to tears hearing it. A mother was told that her very sick baby was not going to survive and that the kindest thing would be to remove her breathing tube and let her die, but the mother would not countenance it. Romana spent time with the mother; in talking to her, it emerged that she was devastated that she had not had the opportunity to breastfeed her child and give her nourishment.

'She felt that she had failed her,' Romana told me. 'In Islam, we are told that we should attempt to nurse our babies, and this mother felt that she was failing in her duty as a mother and as a Muslim.'

Romana spoke to the doctors about the mother's concerns, and they formulated a plan so that when the baby's breathing tube was removed, she would be put on to her mother's breast so that she could squeeze some drops of breast milk on to her lips.

It seemed to me as I spoke to Romana that here, in the chaplaincy team, was the missing link. A trusted person who a family could open up to about concerns they felt they could not share with anyone else, concerns that might actually be the main reason for the breakdown in the communication and the resistance to medical advice.

I wanted to understand more about the role played by hospital chaplains, and how they work with healthcare professionals and families. This whole part of hospital life had not been on my radar until after Daisy had died.

I contacted Nigel, a retired hospital chaplain from Newcastle, to find out more. He told me the word 'chaplaincy' brings with it a lot of baggage that can be a barrier to both families and clinicians engaging in what they do and the support they can offer.

'Hospital chaplains will often have a huge hurdle to overcome to be able to fully engage with families,' he told me. 'Often people have little understanding of why we are there or what we do. They think we'll come in very heavy-handed with religious doctrine, and that may be off-putting to them.'

In fact, as Nigel pointed out, NHS guidance around chaplaincy support is very clear that they are there for people of all faiths and none.

Nigel confirmed how his role, just as Romana had explained, was to try to create a space in which people could genuinely be themselves. To articulate the concerns and feelings that they might be afraid to say to the nurses or the doctors, worried that they may be judged or their concerns seen as trivial. And, if necessary, help to communicate those concerns to the clinicians.

It really struck me, speaking to both Romana and Nigel, that here was an important bridge to humanise conversations. Chaplaincy services give parents space and support so that they feel that they have a voice when speaking to clinicians. An opportunity to articulate their feelings without feeling judged. Sometimes the central concern that causes the disagreement of the parents is wrapped up in their beliefs and tenets of faith. But sometimes it's simply because the family is just overwhelmed, being bombarded on all sides with multiple opinions so that they find themselves in a quandary about what is the right thing to do for their child. And chaplains can act as a bridge between their clinical colleagues and parents in order to develop trust and understanding on both sides, potentially preventing the escalation of disputes into conflicts.

Prior to writing this book, it wouldn't have occurred to me to go and chat to someone in the chaplaincy team about how I was feeling or to ask them to come along to a difficult meeting. Why should I? Daisy was nominally down on her patient information as a baptised Catholic, but my concerns were not centred around any beliefs based on faith (or lack thereof), so it didn't seem like a natural place to gravitate towards. But it's so evident in just speaking to two chaplains that they do have a role to play in helping to advocate, to be a non-judgemental, independent person who can intervene with clinicians to explain a parent's viewpoint. And sometimes to help clinicians speak to parents.

By sitting with my children when I could not be there with them, Romana was supporting me in a way that had nothing to do with faith. It was a human act, an expression of empathy, when I was facing the worst thing a parent could ever face and watching my beloved child take her last breath.

As always, it's not about the role or which department someone is from, their experience or even their faith; it's about humanity and empathy and taking the time to listen.

There is no doubt, however, that parents caring for children with medical complexity carry with them a weight of responsibility and a burden of choice in making the right decision for their child. Framed as what is in their child's 'best interests', it leaves parents with a binary choice – their child lives or their child dies – and hinges on what ultimately constitutes an acceptable quality of life.

CHAPTER 18

Best Interests

FOUR-YEAR-OLD TAFIDA RAQEEB woke her parents one morning in February 2019 complaining that she had a headache. Unbeknownst to Tafida's parents, she had a malformation of the blood vessels in her brain, and these had suddenly ruptured.

She was taken to the hospital and put on a ventilator. After numerous tests, Tafida's parents were informed that she had no awareness or chance of recovery and any further treatment would be futile.

Tafida's parents, both of whom are devout Muslims, refused to accept the doctor's recommendation that removing life-sustaining treatment was in their daughter's best interests. The found a hospital in Italy prepared to perform tracheostomy surgery on Tafida with the hope that she could be weaned off ventilation and ultimately be cared for at home by her parents and trained carers.

A legal challenge ensued as both parties disagreed on what they believed was in the little girl's best interests. Turning to the Islamic Council of Europe, Tafida's mother obtained a fatwa, an opinion on the position in the framework of Islamic Law. It stated that 'it is absolutely impermissible for the parents, or anyone else, to give consent for the removal of the life-supporting machine from their child mentioned'.[1]

---

1   Islamic Council of Europe (2019) 'Case of Tafida Raqeeb – press release. The High Court of Justice agrees with the Islamic Council of Europe on the sanctity of life.' https://iceurope.org/case-of-tafida-raqeeb-press-release

When I spoke to Romana, the Muslim chaplain, she explained that there are guidelines within Islam to support both parents and professionals in these situations. These guidelines can be open to a wide range of interpretations.[2] However, in the eyes of Tafida's parents, any arguments around what was in her best interests were not valid because, as far as they were concerned, within the context of their faith, withdrawing life support would mean killing Tafida.[3]

In his judgement,[4] the judge presiding over the case concluded that while there were 'substantial factors' that supported the case brought by the hospital trust caring for Tafida, he also felt that there were factors that tipped the balance in favour of the parents' request. There was considerable discussion about whether Tafida could feel pain or had an awareness of what was happening to her.

In summing up, the judge commented that 'where there is an absence of clear facts regarding pain or awareness of suffering' – as there was in this case – 'the answer to the objective best interests tests must be looked for in subjective or highly value-laden ethical, moral or religious factors extrinsic to the child'. Such factors include futility, 'dignity, the meaning of life and the principle of the sanctity of life'.

He acknowledged that such factors may 'mean different things to different people in a diverse, multicultural, multifaith society'.

The hospital trust had conceded that transferring Tafida to Italy came with minimal risk (unlike in Alta Fixsler's case where it was perceived that a transfer to an Israeli hospital would cause her further pain and distress). The judge therefore ruled that removing Tafida's life support was not in her best interests and that she *could* be safely transported to Italy 'with little or no impact on her welfare'.

In his discussion on best interests and the religious and cultural

---

2   Mohiuddin, A., Suleman, M., Rasheed, S. and Padela, A.I. (2020) 'When can Muslims withdraw or withhold life support? A narrative review of Islamic juridical rulings.' *Global Bioethics* 31, 1, 29–46.

3   Islamic21C.com (2019) 'Tafida Raqeeb: Is it Islamically permissible to switch off her life support?' https://www.islam21c.com/current-affairs/tafida-raqeeb-is-it-islamically-permissible-to-switch-off-her-life-support

4   *Tafida Raqeeb v Barts NHS Foundation Trust and Others* [2019] EWHC 2531 (Admin) and [2019] EWHC 2530 (Fam).

influences that guided the parents and led to the disagreement with the clinical opinions, he stated that 'the best interests of every child include an expectation that difficult decisions affecting the length and quality of the child's life will be taken for the child by a parent in the exercise of their parental responsibility'.[5]

Tafida was subsequently taken by her parents, with costs borne by them, to a hospital in Italy, where surgery was performed to form a permanent tracheostomy to support her breathing and a gastrostomy to support her nutrition.

Tafida's case was discussed as part of the evidence in Alta Fixsler's case in order to demonstrate that while the situations of the two children appear on the surface to be quite similar, it's clear that there are contrasts and points of differentiation which go some way to explain the differing outcomes.[6]

In Tafida's case, there were uncertainties around whether she was in pain or could feel pain (whereas in Alta's case her clinicians felt very strongly that she was experiencing pain). Tafida's life expectancy (if she was transferred to Italy for the proposed treatment) could potentially be between ten and twenty years, and as she was five when her brain injury occurred, she already had some awareness of the faith in which she was being brought up. This again was in stark contrast to Alta's situation: she was born prematurely, suffering a catastrophic brain injury at birth; she had never left hospital – it was all she knew, if indeed she had awareness of her surroundings.

The similarities and differences in the two cases and the very different outcomes demonstrate how every case like this can only be judged on its unique, individual merits.

---

5   Nottingham, E. (2019) 'Tafida Raqeeb judgment summary: Continuation of life-sustaining treatment in Italy held to be child's best interests.' Transparency Project. https://transparencyproject.org.uk/tafida-raqeeb-judgment-summary-continuation-of-life-sustaining-treatment-in-italy-held-to-be-in-childs-best-interests

6   *Fixsler v Manchester University NHS Foundation Trust* [2021] EWCA Civ 1018. www.judiciary.uk/wp-content/uploads/2021/07/Fixsler-v-Manchester-University-NHS-Foundation-Trust-.pdf

Tafida's case came at the end of a stream of what seemed to be very similar high-profile cases. Each pitted parent against hospital trusts, with disagreements on clinical decisions and recommendations about a very poorly child, particularly around breathing support and access to specialist treatment. In each situation, the judge considered the evidence presented based on whether it was in the child's 'best interests'.

No wonder these cases are so difficult and garner such huge media attention. When parents are asked to consider what is in our child's best interests, we make a value judgement on what we believe is right for them, within the framework of our own experience, beliefs and values as parents.

Over and over, I have heard parents of some of the sickest children say 'where there's life there's hope', and in each of these cases there was a glimmer of hope that treatment, even if it was long-term ventilation with no chance of neurological improvement, was, for the parents, a better option than death. That's what makes these cases so difficult and heartrendingly impossible. It goes to the heart of a parent's desire to do 'anything for my child'.

For some parents, this will be to accept the most extreme of odds and the prospect of a life of constant caring for a child who might never respond to them. For others, it will be to accept the advice of the clinicians to end life-sustaining treatment.

Doctors might consider further treatment to be 'futile' or 'potentially inappropriate',[7] whereas some parents want treatment to continue in the hope, however remote, that they may see some improvement in their child's condition. There is inherent emotion in these positions with no right or wrong answer, just agonising decisions and sometimes long and protracted court cases which place families and clinicians in the spotlight. In the six months that Charlie Gard's parents campaigned for him to be allowed to

---

7   Wilkinson, D. (2017) 'Debate response: Charlie Gard, interests and justice – an alternative view.' Journal of Medical Ethics Blog, 26 April. https://blogs.bmj.com/medical-ethics/2017/04/26/debate-reponse-charlie-gard-interests-and-justice-an-alternative-view

be taken to the USA for experimental treatment, Charlie was in an intensive care unit, attached to a ventilator, while the debate on what was in his best interests continued around him.

Should doctors even be talking about 'best interests' in their conversations with parents? Do they really know what they mean when they use this term? An ethicist told me recently that he has increasingly tried to counsel paediatricians against talking about 'best interests' with parents, recommending instead that doctors talk to the parents and try to work out together what is the best way of caring for the child. Exploring what would help them, trying to avoid things that may do more harm than good.

Following these cases, and other less high-profile ones, some ethicists have begun to discuss whether a value judgement of a child's 'best interests' is appropriate in these scenarios. As the Australian philosopher and bioethicist Julian Savalescu states:

> Best interests apply across a number of decisions around children, for example in family law cases, when two parents might reasonably disagree about decisions affecting a child the court is asked to choose which option is in the child's best interests: which on the balance of probabilities will lead to the best outcomes. However, in a case involving limitation of life prolonging treatment, one option ends the life of the child.[8]

So the question then becomes: is it appropriate to decide what is in the best interests of a very sick child when one of the options on the table is their death? Even if the child is believed to be in pain or discomfort, then some parents may be prepared to accept a symptom care regimen with complex analgesia to manage that pain over their child's death.

In fact, framing decisions and conversations around 'best interests' has the potential to further stir up conflict. Parents can

8   Savulescu, J. (2017) 'Debate: The fiction of an interest in death? Justice for Charlie Gard.' Journal of Medical Ethics Blog, 26 April. https://blogs.bmj. com/medical-ethics/2017/04/26/debate-the-fiction-of-an-interest-in-death-justice-for-charlie-gard

potentially feel aggrieved that doctors claim to know better than the parents what is best for their child. And making a determination about best interests in a courtroom will automatically run contrary to the views of the parents. It sets them up in opposition to their child's doctors, fuelling a narrative of a battle to be won or lost.

Is there another approach to how decisions could be made about a child's treatment where there is disagreement with professionals?

Professor Dominic Wilkinson argues that there is an 'elephant in the room' in most of the cases concerning disagreements between parents and clinicians about the care for a minimally conscious child, and that is the question of available resources.[9]

While you cannot put a price on the life of a child, what happens when giving life-sustaining treatment and care to one child means that another child is denied that care?

We experienced many occasions when Daisy needed a paediatric intensive care bed but none was available. I learned very early on that it's not about the bed space; it's about the availability of the highly trained, specialist staff and equipment needed to care for the child in that bed. There are a finite number of intensive care beds in the UK, and every day intensive care consultants have to make a decision about who can have the next available bed. We had numerous reviews by the 'exceptional circumstances' committee of our clinical commissioning group to decide whether they would fund a drug or treatment that could improve Daisy's quality of life. At one point, with a fridge full of TPN, a room full of various drugs and equipment and a home that looked like an extension of a hospital high-dependency unit, I was told, 'Your daughter is the most expensive child in the borough.' That investment was keeping my child alive and allowing her to have an acceptable quality of life in terms that were meaningful to us and her.

As Professor Wilkinson postulates in the same paper:

9 Cameron, J., Savulescu, J. and Wilkinson, D. (2022) 'Raqeeb, Haastrup, and Evans: Seeking consistency through a distributive justice-based approach to limitation of treatment in the context of dispute.' *Journal of Law, Medicine & Ethics* 50, 1, 169–180.

While the question of whether treatment was in the best interests of the children in the cases discussed is extremely difficult, the decisions by the NHS trusts not to offer long-term mechanical ventilation appears much more clear-cut when viewed in terms of resources.

It's horrible, isn't it? The reality is that there are just not enough specialist resources or funding to care for everyone, and clinicians have to make very tough decisions on who gets the bed space, who gets the funding for a home care package for ventilation support, who gets the specialist drug treatment...weighing this up against every single child who needs treatment.

But some ethicists are now arguing that a 'distributive justice' approach to these complex cases is a more relevant measure than 'best interests'.

Distributive justice recognises the context in which decisions are made. It avoids making judgements about the value of human life and focuses instead on the competing demands on the limited healthcare resources available at the time. This approach has the potential, in the view of some ethicists, to move the narrative away from a binary discussion on whether a life is worth living to relative conversations around the value of life and the availability of resources to support that life.

Professor Wilkinson goes on to explain:

Focusing on the appropriate use of resources may change the process according to which hospitals may intervene in parental decisions to seek treatment elsewhere. The distributive justice approach would recognise that the resources available to an NHS Trust are limited and that it may not be appropriate to expend these on long term mechanical ventilation of a child who experiences no apparent enjoyment from life. But this alternative approach may also clarify that if the parents are able to find an alternative means of accessing mechanical ventilation, there may no longer be a strong reason to prevent the child from accessing it.

But as a bereaved parent recently told me, what about the cases where a child is ventilated and stabilised but the parents then have to fight and fight for every element of care and support for the rest of the child's life? The child's life has been saved, but lack of funds and social care support puts their life at risk as their exhausted parents struggle to care for them...at the cost of their health and the potential detrimental impact on the wider family. Resources need to be available to support the child and family for the rest of their life, potentially way into adulthood.

These are all value-based decisions, rooted in complexity. Parents need support to make decisions for their child; they need recommendations and guidance from the doctors treating their child. In the same vein, they need to know that their role as advocates and parents is valued. There is a balance to be struck between objectively working out what is in a child's best interests and also ensuring parents feel both validated and supported. Doctors, for all their training and experience, are (for the most part) not experts in ethical evaluation, and they need to be careful not to make recommendations for children based on their own personal values.

In many cases, there is no single right answer (but there can be wrong answers). There are just difficult decisions, and these cannot and should not be made on the spur of the moment and without an ongoing dialogue with parents. Wishes around resuscitation, for example, should be discussed well in advance of a decision being needed, and these conversations should take place in an appropriate setting.

I was used to discussing my resuscitation wishes for Daisy. Whenever we went to the hospice for a respite stay, this was a standard question that was asked on admission. My response was always the same – full active resuscitation, qualified with the statement 'I'll know when the time is right not to attempt resuscitation'. And I did.

This is something that my friend Saira has spent a lot of time thinking about. She is very clear that there should be no more invasive treatment for her daughter Samara, except that which maintains her quality of life and controls her symptoms.

We can't define what constitutes an acceptable quality of life. As individuals, we have our own views, based on our own experience on what that means for us. As parents, we are entrusted with deciding what that means for our child. We face decisions that no parent should ever have to make. We have to second-guess what we believe our child would want us to do, within the framework of our own system of values and beliefs, and within the guidelines of the prevailing law and what is medically possible.

It's complex – beyond complex. These decisions are agonising for parents, patients and clinicians alike. There are no winners, just the sort of ethical dilemma that any average person hopes they never have to face in their lifetime. There will be more and more of these conversations and difficult decisions, and possibly more high-profile court cases as medicine is able to do more to sustain life and clinicians are faced with the perennial question: 'Just because we can, does it mean we should?'

In our desire to ensure parents are involved and have their say in what they want for their child, are we also in danger of burdening them with an overwhelming responsibility? There's a term in medical ethics called 'abandoning someone to their own autonomy'. I learned it when speaking to a friend who also happens to be a doctor interested in this area.[10]

Patient autonomy, as I explained previously, is about helping patients (or parents of patients) make reasoned choices.

As my doctor friend explained to me, a generation ago we had a 'paternalistic' approach to medicine, one where 'doctor knows best' and patients did not question their judgement. Now the pendulum has swung the other way, where patients have more autonomy in the choices they make for their body. But has it swung too far? Are there times when parents have been 'abandoned to their autonomy'? Given options and left to make their own choices for their child.

As he explained this concept to me, my head filled with countless examples of where this had happened in caring for Daisy: 'We

---

10 He wishes to remain anonymous.

can try this med and it may do this, or we could try that – what do you want to do?' Over and over, it felt that the onus of trying to make the right decision for my child fell on our shoulders as parents; no one would tell us what to do – just give us options. The most extreme example was when Daisy was at end of life, on the intensive care ward. The intensive care consultant who was attending that day didn't know Daisy or me. After Daisy's cardiac arrest, she spoke to me and said that they could keep resuscitating, they could try starting kidney dialysis...what did I want to do?

It was fortunate that I had already had many years to think about what to do, that I knew in my head what the right thing to do would be. Even though it went against my instinct as a mother, it was the right thing for Daisy.

Romana, the Muslim chaplain I interviewed, also expressed her unease about this shift. She was concerned that many of the conflicts she witnesses in her work around decision making for a child at end of life stem from our Western medicine approach to place the burden of decision making on the child's family. She can see it's an unbearable burden, to ask a parent to make the final decision on what is essentially a binary choice – whether their child will live or die.

There's no doubt that this pressure on parents to be the final arbiters of their child's fate must prolong the process as parents wrestle with the decision, going back to questions of faith, or whether they are giving up on their child, swayed by the opinions of others and who they might be letting down in making what could be perceived to be the 'wrong' choice. Many of these parents have just landed in the world of complex needs; they have not journeyed in the same way that those who have walked this path for years have. I had time to adjust, I had time with my daughter, and in my head the decision was very clear. But I can't imagine trying to make decisions about whether or not to continue with Daisy's life support when she was a baby and I was just navigating my way in this world.

Parents need support with decision making to make informed decisions about their child's treatment, and that relies on a relationship of trust between clinicians and parents. By abandoning parents to make their own decisions, however well intentioned, we open up the potential for a breakdown of trust where parents feel they must shop for second opinions or resort to Dr Google to work out what's best for their child.

Clinicians should feel that they are in control and are supporting parents in making the right decision for their child, in doing what's best for them. Back to Professor Wilkinson again – he has described a 'grey zone' involved in navigating end-of-life care for critically ill children. His work focuses on the ethical dilemmas faced by clinicians on when it is appropriate to resuscitate a premature baby, but it has relevance to decisions around the care of a child with complex medical needs.

The grey zone lies in the space between an upper threshold of care involving clear-cut decisions to resuscitate and a lower threshold where further intervention is deemed futile. The boundaries of the zones are defined by clinical evidence which guides decision making, and the grey zone falls in the middle where there is uncertainty.

Writing about these issues,[11] Wilkinson describes the grey zone as 'a set of clinical situations in which resuscitation and intensive care will be provided to newborn infants if parents so wish, or will be withheld/withdrawn (and palliative care provided) if parents choose'.

It's a tough one, because the onus is on the parents to decide. I'm not the expert here, but these sorts of decisions and discussions around whether or not to resuscitate happen frequently in the neonatal situation, but what about further down the line? When it's no longer about prematurity?

That's where (excuse the pun here) decision making really does become grey. I have found myself going down an ethics rabbit hole

---

11 Wilkinson, D. (2016) 'Who Should Decide for Critically Ill Neonates and How? The Grey Zone in Neonatal Treatment Decisions.' In R. McDougall, C. Delany and L. Gillam (eds) *When Doctors and Parents Disagree: Ethics, Paediatrics and the Zone of Parental Discretion.* Sydney: The Federation Press.

with this one – beyond the grey zone, a 'zone of parental discretion' (ZPD) has been described which is 'the ethically protected space where parents may legitimately make decisions for their children, even if the decisions are sub-optimal for those children'.[12] This ZPD moves beyond decisions around whether or not to resuscitate and into wider decisions around treatment beyond the neonatal stage.

And that ZPD and where its boundaries lie are at the heart of whether or not parents and clinicians can reach agreement on the right course of action for the child at the centre.

The ethical theory is fascinating, but in the same way as I became fascinated by genetics and understanding as much as possible about Daisy's condition, it can be a distraction. I can't imagine many clinicians would be faced with a situation around continuing care and think, 'Ah, yes, we're in the zone of parental discretion here...' There's a huge amount of subjectivity and prior experience that comes with these scenarios.

Doctors and parents need help to navigate these difficult ethical decisions, because, ultimately, every situation is unique. Just because Daisy had Costello syndrome, it didn't mean that we were able to predict how she would develop or respond. Parents have value systems and views that differ from those of the parents caring for the child in the next bed. But they need support to understand how to work their way through the unbelievably complex and emotional decisions they have to make on behalf of their child. To help them stand back and try to objectively make decisions that no parent should ever be expected to make.

Once again it comes down to communication, to building trust, to collaboration and also, perhaps, to clinicians swinging the pendulum back a little bit. We are the experts on our child, but there is a reason doctors studied for years at medical school, and together we should be able to work as a team.

12   Wilkinson, D. (2016) 'Who Should Decide for Critically Ill Neonates and How? The Grey Zone in Neonatal Treatment Decisions.' In R. McDougall, C. Delany and L. Gillam (eds) *When Doctors and Parents Disagree: Ethics, Paediatrics and the Zone of Parental Discretion.* Sydney: The Federation Press.

I wonder if I was unusual. I needed 'team Daisy' around me to help me make decisions. I knew that, as her mum, there would always be an emotional element, but I needed to be able to stand back and try to think about what was the right thing for Daisy. 'Anything for my child' isn't always the right thing for my child. I knew nothing about clinical ethics when Daisy was alive, apart from my awareness of this mysterious group who (as I mistakenly thought) could make life or death decisions about my child. Parents have access to more and more information on the choices available than ever, so maybe it's time for clinicians to help with that education, bringing them into the fold.

I struggled with the culture of doctors always giving me choices and not helping me work out what was the best one. I would sometimes say to them, 'If it was your child, what would you do?' I know it's unfair, but sometimes you just have to push back, and in pushing back, that can also humanise the conversation, demystifying the process and creating a better balance between autonomy and advice.

So how can we support professionals and parents in having these difficult conversations? I discussed chaplaincy services in Chapter 17, but what other recourse is there for parents when trust breaks down and parents and clinicians are unable to reach consensus?

Who can help everyone involved try to see the wood for the trees and make the best decision for the child (even if it might be the worst thing you ever have to do as a parent)?

◇ CHAPTER 19 ◇

Call It by Its Name

'WE NEED TO ACKNOWLEDGE IT, call it by its name.' I was speaking to Dr Esse Menson, a paediatrician who now works full-time as a mediator for the Medical Mediation Foundation (MMF) in the UK. The 'it' she was referring to is conflict. In her view, professionals need to move away from labelling families caring for children as 'difficult' or a 'problem' when conflict occurs. They need to acknowledge that communication has broken down, and the work then needs start in order to restore it.

The MMF was founded in 2010 by former BBC health journalist Sarah Barclay. Sarah had covered the high-profile case of a young leukaemia patient called Jaymee Bowen – referred to in the courts at the time as 'Child B' – for a *Panorama* documentary and subsequently wrote a book about the case.

Jaymee Bowen's story is harrowing and all too familiar: a child for whom all treatment options had run out; a father determined to leave no stone unturned, unwilling to accept that palliative care was the only option available for his child. He scoured the world looking for doctors who might offer an alternative and persuaded an oncologist who specialised in treating adults to take on his daughter's care, against the advice of her clinicians.

When his local health authority refused to fund a second bone marrow transplant for his daughter (her oncologists had advised against it, recommending symptom management instead), Jaymee's father launched a high-profile court case to challenge this decision, claiming that it was based on NHS rationing. Ultimately, a private doctor stepped in to pay for Jaymee's treatment (she never did have the transplant and instead received further chemo and what, at the time, was experimental and unproven treatment) and she lived for another year.

A review of the case highlighted a number of recommendations,[1] one of the most significant being a call for decision makers to explain the reasons behind decisions, show that these are relevant and give the patient (or, in this case, the parent) an opportunity to appeal:

> The reason for emphasising the need to improve the process of decision making is that cases of this kind are always likely to generate debate and disagreement. What therefore matters is to structure the debate to enable different points of view to be articulated; to promote transparency and consistency in decision making; and to build trust, confidence, and legitimacy in the process. In the longer term, these characteristics of due process in decision making should enhance public understanding of choices in health care and promote more informed discussion of the issues. These lessons need to be acted on by health authorities and primary care groups.[2]

Through her work on this story and other similar ones, Sarah became increasingly interested in looking at the role good communication and listening skills play in resolving the breakdown of relationships between clinicians and families. Looking back at the press coverage, it's clear that central to the case is a disagreement between a parent and his daughter's clinicians about how far to go in treating Jaymee and what was in her best interests as a terminally ill child.

Sarah decided to leave journalism and founded the MMF in

1   Ham, C. (1999) 'Tragic choices in health care: Lessons from the Child B case.' *BMJ* 319, 7219, 1258–1261. doi:10.1136/bmj.319.7219.1258
2   Ham, C. (1999) 'Tragic choices in health care: Lessons from the Child B case.' *BMJ* 319, 7219, 1258–1261. doi:10.1136/bmj.319.7219.1258

order to focus her time on helping families resolve disagreements with clinicians.

The foundation offers independent mediation services for families and clinicians where trust and communication has broken down so that they can move forward and potentially avoid the situation escalating to the family court. As Sarah commented in an interview with *The Guardian*: 'A trained mediator can't decide what is best, but he or she can make sure that everyone is heard and seek a resolution with as little collateral damage as possible.'[3]

But as she told me:

> There will always be cases which, rightly, need to be decided by the courts. There are other cases where mediation can prevent that from happening. And even before that, our focus is on trying to prevent these disagreements becoming conflicts in the first place.

Over the past decade, the MMF has delivered training programmes to clinicians in a number of hospital trusts, sharing strategies and approaches to help staff at all levels de-escalate conflict and prevent disputes. It's not rocket science really; the training focuses on the fundamentals of how clinical staff communicate to parents and how this can impact behaviour. The aim is to create a mindset shift, from labelling a 'problem parent' to thinking about what has caused that parent to respond to the situation in the way they have. In a half-day session, Sarah, Esse and their colleagues take doctors, nurses and other health professionals on a journey where they get to feel what it's like to be on the other side of the hospital bed. I've observed a few of these sessions now, and there are always some clear lightbulb moments as the attendees begin to understand the lived experience of the parents they are speaking to on a day-to-day basis, and how these interactions can impact behaviours.

As any childcare expert will tell you, behaviour is always rooted

---

3   Roberts, Y. (2014) 'Now there's a chance for families to avoid their own Ashya King anguish.' *The Observer*, 7 September. www.theguardian.com/society/2014/sep/07/how-mediation-prevent-repeat-ashya-king-case-nhs

in experience, and turning criticism to empathy and making the time to listen can help de-escalate a situation.

'It's not easy,' Sarah told me, 'but supporting health professionals to stand in the shoes of the parents, to understand the parents' lived experience, helping clinicians to think about the impact of their words and giving them the skills and confidence to have conversations differently can help disagreements from becoming conflicts.'

This shift in communication takes time and a requires a huge cultural change – our UK healthcare system is very much rooted in the philosophy of 'doctor knows best', and while this approach is changing and there is an increased recognition of the need for co-production, collaboration and understanding a patient's lived experience, this change can take time to be embedded. Humanising how we communicate, asking parents what they want to be called (back to the 'Don't call me mum' theme again), listening and taking time to understand what has brought a parent to this point are all ways to make this happen. Not many professionals get the chance to step into the family's world; we come into theirs most of the time – the controlled situation of the ward or the outpatient clinic. I would always make a point of bringing a picture of Daisy to meetings or of talking specifically about our life at home in order to bring professionals into our lives so they could see Daisy not just as a patient but as a little girl, part of a family.

'Not every case can be mediated, and that's for a number of different reasons. Sometimes it's because parties are unwilling or unable to be open to another viewpoint. Sometimes what the family want and what the clinicians believe is acceptable leaves very little mediatable territory, and try as we may, it's not going to happen,' Sarah told me, 'but my long-term aim is to get to a point where, by supporting clinicians to understand how to avoid or de-escalate conflict by building empathetic communication, they will be able to resolve disagreements without the need for more formal processes such as mediation.'

Karina's story

I sat on the press bench of the coroner's court and looked at the woman in front of me. It was day three of the hearing into the death of her beloved first-born child, Melody. The woman was Karina, Melody's mum. She was hunched up, rocking gently; every now and then, she would shake her head in disagreement at what she was hearing, or nod in approval. Her pain was palpable.

I'd known Karina from stays on the gastro ward at Great Ormond Street Hospital. I remember a mutual friend telling me I should meet her because our girls were so very similar. She was right: while they had different diagnoses – Melody was diagnosed with Rett syndrome – Melody was also TPN dependent and, like Daisy, she also had lots of other issues going on that were not in the standard textbook for her syndrome.

Karina and I knew of each other, but we didn't really get to know each other until I began my work for this book. I knew that our lives had taken very different paths, and we had taken very different approaches to dealing with the conflicts that arose as we tried to advocate for our daughters.

What I knew about Melody came mainly through press reports, posted on the family's public Facebook page.[4] There had been a breakdown in the family's relationship with their children's hospice, and social services had become involved,[5] and then a couple of years later, I began to see press reports and Facebook updates about legal action Karina and her husband were taking as a different specialist hospital that now managed Melody's care had brought in social services to assess whether Melody should be taken into foster care.[6]

4   'Melody In Mind.' Facebook. www.facebook.com/Melodyinmind
5   Downey, A. (2016) 'New Addington mum, Karina Driscoll, "treated like a criminal" after Shooting Star Chase hospice wrongly alleged she abused her daughter Melody.' *Sutton & Croydon Guardian*, 14 September. www.yourlocalguardian.co.uk/news/14741771.mum-treated-like-criminal-hospice-wrongly-alleged-abused-seriously-ill-daughter
6   Mackintosh, T. (2018) 'Melody Driscoll: Croydon Council bid for wardship fails.' BBC News, 17 April. www.bbc.co.uk/news/uk-england-london-43386929

All of this information was in the public domain, and as I sat on the sidelines, I asked myself what had happened for this family to find themselves turning to the media to raise awareness of what was going on? How had things become so bad that social services were accusing Karina of fabricating the severity of Melody's illness and her need for continuous pain medication?

Melody died in July 2018. Her death was not the controlled, pain-free death that I felt I was able to give Daisy. At Melody's end of life, it seems that Karina was barely communicating with the team caring for her daughter. There was a complete breakdown of trust, and Karina had been accused by the consultant responsible for safeguarding at the hospital trust of lying about the severity of her daughter's symptoms.[7]

Fabricated induced illness (FII) is the term for the condition previously referred to as Munchausen's syndrome by proxy. FII is a rare form of child abuse. The NHS website describes it as a situation when a parent or carer, usually the child's biological mother, exaggerates or deliberately causes symptoms of illness in the child.[8]

More recently, however, guidance to support healthcare professionals to be alert to FII has been expanded to include perplexing presentations and medically unexplained symptoms. That's an interesting one: how does that label fit with the comment that was made to me when Daisy was a baby that 'this level of complexity is academic guesswork'? Unexplained symptoms are a huge part of medicine, after all – just because a doctor doesn't understand something doesn't mean it doesn't exist. And surely, in a world where children are outliving their prognoses and surviving longer, often showing new and unexplained symptoms, is this catch-all label a valid tool to accuse parents of abuse?

The official guidance from the Royal College of Paediatric and

7   Hockaday, J. (2021) 'Mum demands answers after doctor "accused her of faking daughter's symptoms"'. *Metro*, 6 May https://metro.co.uk/2021/05/06/mum-demands-probe-after-doctor-accused-her-of-faking-daughters-symptoms-14523402

8   NHS (n.d.) 'Fabricated or induced illness.' www.nhs.uk/mental-health/conditions/fabricated-or-induced-illness

Child Health (RCPCH),[9] which aims to support clinicians, puts FII and perplexing presentations into the same category, and this can be misleading. In other words, the guidelines to help clinicians confronted with very rare incidences of abuse (FII) are presented alongside potential scenarios where anxious parents are requesting more support to find out what is going on with their child. Surely this will lead to more false positives, breaking down trust and communication between clinicians and parents?

There are genuine and thankfully rare cases where parents have fabricated their child's illness, causing them to have lifelong disabilities and even causing their death. I remember when Daisy was first a patient on a neurology ward at Great Ormond Street Hospital, a new protocol had just been put in place to ensure that all specialist formula milks were kept in locked fridges. Earlier that year, a mother on that same ward had been arrested and imprisoned as it had been found that she was adding salt to her son's formula, and this had caused his death.[10]

Is there a bias in the official guidance towards some parents caring for medically complex children that drives clinicians to think they are fabricating their symptoms? Some paediatricians claim they are seeing more and more FII cases in their practice. Dr Alison Steele, officer for child protection and safeguarding at the RCPCH and consultant paediatrician at Great Ormond Street Hospital, has commented in the media, saying, 'Certainly when you talk to designated doctors up and down the country they are dealing regularly with these sorts of issues and cases.'[11]

Conversely, one doctor who specialises in caring for children

---

9 Royal College of Paediatrics and Child Health (2022) 'Perplexing Presentations (PP)/Fabricated or Induced Illness (FII) in children – guidance.' Child Protection Portal. https://childprotection.rcpch.ac.uk/resources/perplexing-presentations-and-fii

10 Dyer, C. (2005) 'Mother found guilty in case of fabricated illness.' *BMJ 330*, 7490, 497. www.ncbi.nlm.nih.gov/pmc/articles/PMC552836

11 PA News Agency (2001) 'Fabricated illness in children "much more common" than previously thought.' *Helensburgh Advertiser*, 2 March. www.helensburghadvertiser.co.uk/news/national-news/19130115.fabricated-illness-children-much-common-previously-thought

with medical complexity at a large children's hospital told me (on condition of anonymity), 'There's no such thing as FII in medically complex kids (or if there is, it's very rare), but what we do see is anxious and stressed parents trying to support their children.'

Some doctors believe that 'Dr Google' is contributing to anxiety in parents – apparently, it's called *cyberchondria*. Parents caring for medically complex children are not doctors, but we need to have a level of knowledge about our child, their baselines, their responses, that doctors cannot be expected to have. And when it comes to Dr Google, a new study suggests that 'using online resources to research symptoms may not be harmful after all – and could even lead to modest improvements in diagnosis'.[12]

Living with Daisy 24/7, I noticed subtle things, I tuned in to her world, and I needed our clinicians to listen to me and trust me when I told them that I thought something was not right. FII exists, and it's very real and also very, very rare. For some parents caring for children with medical complexity, however, it has the potential to be used as a way of controlling them when trust breaks down and conflict occurs. An accusation of FII is the fastest way of removing a parent's ability to advocate for their child.

Melody spent most of her life as a hospital inpatient, with very few extended periods at home. She became sicker and sicker, and management of her pain became more and more difficult. Melody began to have excruciating pain episodes which seemed unrelated to her main Rett syndrome diagnosis. By this point, she was under the care of the hospital palliative team, having been an inpatient for months. A plan was made to let her come home with a background infusion of morphine and ketamine to help manage her pain. The intention was to wean Melody off these pain meds once she was stable, and Karina agreed to this. But disagreements soon began

---

12   *Irish Times* (2021) 'Dr Google: Searching your symptoms may not be such a bad idea after all.' Health, 30 March. www.irishtimes.com/life-and-style/health-family/dr-google-searching-your-symptoms-may-not-be-such-a-bad-idea-after-all-1.4523915

between Karina and the doctors over when and how to reduce Melody's pain medication.[13]

A specialist procedure to remove a gallstone resulted in perforation of Melody's bowel, and she developed acute pancreatitis. Melody became desperately ill, and the intensive care doctors struggled to stabilise her. Melody died weeks later of multiple organ failure and gastrointestinal haemorrhage. During the coroner's inquest, Melody's parents alleged that the actions of the clinicians during this time, including their continued efforts to reduce her pain medication, reduced her quality of life and contributed to her death.[14]

The family's barrister told the inquest that Melody's parents were 'haunted by the belief that Melody died in pain because she was not listened to'.[15]

In press reports following the inquest, Karina claimed that the hospital treating Melody had a 'we know best attitude' and that she was not listened to. During the inquest, the court was shown an email in which one doctor told another staff member they 'should not pander to this family'.[16]

It's clear from the press coverage of the case and her heartfelt posts on her public Facebook page that Karina has been broken.[17] She is mourning the death of her daughter but lives with the guilt that she let her down in some way. Speaking to the press after the inquest, Karina commented that she and her husband had felt they

13 Hockaday, J. (2021) 'Mum demands answers after doctor "accused her of faking daughter's symptoms"'. *Metro*, 6 May https://metro.co.uk/2021/05/06/mum-demands-probe-after-doctor-accused-her-of-faking-daughters-symptoms-14523402

14 BBC News (2021, 22 March) 'Melody Driscoll: Doctors ignored concerns over seriously ill girl.' www.bbc.co.uk/news/uk-england-london-56489142

15 William, H. (2021) 'Reducing pain medication not a factor in Rett syndrome girl's death: Coroner.' Medscape UK, 1 April. www.medscape.com/viewarticle/948519

16 William, H. (2021) 'Reducing pain medication not a factor in Rett syndrome girl's death: Coroner.' Medscape UK, 1 April. www.medscape.com/viewarticle/948519; BBC News (2021, 1 April) 'Melody Driscoll inquest: Eleven-year-old died of "worst pancreatitis"'. www.bbc.co.uk/news/uk-england-london-56521007

17 'Melody In Mind.' Facebook. www.facebook.com/Melodyinmind

had been branded as 'problematic parents for trying to do the best for their daughter'.[18]

But why should we expect the emotionally and physically exhausted parent to meet the professionals on the same ground? Why can't doctors try to stand in our shoes in order to change the narrative, to advocate and support and understand rather than create a complex web of unanswered questions and accusations?

Where can parents turn when faced with the most complex of decisions about their child, when they feel they are not listened to? I thought about Sarah Barclay's work with the MMF.

When I spoke to Karina, I wanted to know if she had any thoughts on what could have been done to change things. 'Mediation,' she told me. 'I wish we'd had been offered a chance of that.'

I only found out about the existence of mediation services after Daisy died. In fact, mediation is very much in its infancy, and many clinicians still don't understand how it could potentially help.

I had only one formalised way of trying to negotiate a disagreement with clinicians in my time caring for Daisy. Hospital patient advice and liaison services (PALS) were created in 2002 to provide information and on-the-spot help where patients want to resolve a problem without making a formal complaint. Its role is to provide confidential advice, support and reassurance, and to resolve small problems locally. PALS are also allowed to assist with the filing of a formal complaint in addition to their informal resolution powers.

Over the years, I got to know the service very well. I escalated a few concerns through them, and I would frequently ask for their advice and support on situations that we faced. But it struck me that for children like Daisy, with many consultants and hospital admissions, the PALS was not the place to go. There was a limit to how they could help, and our situation was just too complex for them to really help us navigate the difficult conversations and potential communication breakdowns.

---

18 Merrifield, R. (2021) 'Devastated mum brings ashes of tragic daughter, 11, to inquest into her death.' *Mirror*, 1 April. www.mirror.co.uk/news/uk-news/devastated-mum-brings-ashes-tragic-23834528

PALS is not an advocacy service, after all; they can deal with small problems but not big ongoing issues. They're a signposting service and they are also the complaints function for the hospital trust. This means that they are not truly independent: if a parent complains about a clinician, the hospital is essentially investigating themselves. There is no clear recourse to independent advocacy and support for parents who find themselves struggling to hear themselves heard. It's the step before mediation, before communications truly break down, and there's a big gap in how parents are supported in this area.

I navigated my way through it all as best I could, driven, like every parent I have spoken to, by a need to be heard and for my voice to be part of the conversations about my child. I made it work in a way, but in hindsight, I was one of the luckier ones to have found a couple of wonderful consultants who stuck with us and were able to help my voice to be amplified. Not everyone is that lucky.

And, of course, now, with more and more choices and possibilities, with greater focus on parental autonomy, the never-ending question is always there: 'Just because we can, does it mean we should?' What happens when decisions about whether or not to go ahead with a surgery, prescribe a drug, continue treatment get really difficult, when doctors disagree or just struggle with deciding what is the right thing to do for the child?

'It's going to ethics...' It's a comment I've heard from many parents facing huge decisions about the next steps in their child's care and management. What are these mysterious clinical ethics committees? What is their remit, and who are they there to help?

CHAPTER 20

Demystifying Ethics

O VER THE PAST DECADE, the number of clinical ethics committees (CECs) in hospital trusts has multiplied exponentially.
The Covid pandemic saw many new committees formed as clinicians struggled with questions around allocation of intensive care
beds while faced with unprecedented demand for this expensive
resource. CECs provide advice and support on ethical issues arising
from clinical practice and patient care within a healthcare organisation. In fact, some confirm this role as an 'adviser' by calling
themselves clinical ethics advisory groups. No 'official' guidelines
exist for the formation of CECs, and there's no real monitoring
of their outputs. The UK Clinical Ethics Network (UKCEN)[1] is a
national organisation that aims to promote the role of ethics support in clinical practice and attempts to coordinate and promote
the work of ethics committees across the UK. But the reality is that
there is no formal coordination of CECs and their work; they are
voluntary groups, and even their membership can vary.

They exist to provide advice, similar to asking the opinion of a
sub-specialist. It's then up to the clinician whether they will follow
that advice. That's the theory, but the perception and implemen-
tation varies.

In 2020, a judge presiding over a case considering the care
of a child with extremely complex medical needs remarked that

---

1   www.ukcen.net

while the CEC in the treating hospital had reached a consensus on the child's long-term care and medical management, the parents had not been invited to attend or represent their case to the CEC.[2] In other words, where was the opportunity for the parents' voice to be heard when an ethics panel discusses the care of their child?

The UKCEN website states: 'Current practice of most UK CECs does not usually involve patients or their families and carers in the committee's discussion but some committees have considered cases at the request of a patient's family or carer.'[3]

Some CECs involve parents or patient representatives, but their unregulated and inconsistent structure means it's difficult to know when or if parents are asked to be involved in situations where their child's case is being discussed. Or even if parents are aware that their child's case is the subject of an ethics review.

That was certainly the case with me. It was only after Daisy died that I learned that her case had been discussed by an ethics panel. This obviously meant that I was not consulted on my opinion about the huge surgery and ongoing treatment with TPN that were discussed at the review. The surgery went ahead, but what if, as a result of consulting the CEC, Daisy's team had decided not to proceed? I hadn't even been aware that there were concerns that putting Daisy through surgery was the right thing to do. Should this have been discussed with me? In my opinion, yes, it should have been. Learning of the discussions after the event made me feel that I was excluded from conversations. If the clinicians had then told me the surgery was off, what recourse would I have had to present a case for why I believed it should take place?

Even when they are told that their child will be the subject of an ethics review, how do parents feel about it? They may be unaware

---

2   Sokol, D. (2020) 'A wake-up call for clinical ethics committees.' The BMJ Opinion, 27 July. https://blogs.bmj.com/bmj/2020/07/27/daniel-sokol-a-wake-up-call-for-clinical-ethics-committees

3   UKCEN (n.d.) 'Practical guide to clinical ethics support.' www.ukcen.net/education_resources/support_guide/section_a_clinical_ethics_support

or unsure of what that means or what the outcome might signal for their future, something over which they have no control.

What happens at these mysterious ethics panels? How do they function, what do they do, how do they operate?

I have now observed three clinical ethics panel sessions at different hospital trusts; all were virtual meetings thanks to Covid but just as useful in giving an insight into their work.

Each one had a very diverse membership base from faith leaders to retired solicitors. There were, of course, clinicians and nursing staff and, yes, there were patient representatives on each. But I was left with the feeling that, despite their best efforts, these are not independent groups; they are (mainly) aligned to hospital trusts and very much driven by clinicians and for clinicians. The remit seems to be a forum to help clinicians come up with a recommended course of action when faced with complex and ethically challenging decisions about a child's treatment. They support clinicians to try to find some clarity as they wrestle with huge and complex dilemmas.

As an ethicist working with CECs confirmed to me, their role is to provide advice to the clinicians for what to do if they have a disagreement with patients. For example, it might include 'Seek a second opinion', 'Have you thought about mediation?', 'Explore the possibility of compromise', or 'Go to court'. They are not the solution for all conflicts between doctors and families. Their function is to support clinicians, not families.

There are differing viewpoints on whether involving parents in CECs is a good thing. Dominic Wilkinson believes that involving parents in presenting their case would change the nature and remit of CECs.[4] My view is that, in cases of conflict, the CEC is one of a multi-disciplinary approach to resolution. A CEC helps bring clarity to the ethical dilemma, but it does not help in managing complete communications breakdowns between clinicians and parents.

4   Wilkinson, D. and Dunn, M. (2020) 'Must clinical ethics committees involve patients or families in their meetings?' Practical Ethics, 3 August. http://blog. practicalethics.ox.ac.uk/2020/08/must-clinical-ethics-committees-involve-patients-or-families-in-their-meetings

CECs need to sit alongside independent mediation and advocacy in providing a more holistic approach, where everyone's voice is respected and heard, to resolving disputes and conflicts without recourse to the courts.

Preventing disagreements escalating into conflicts starts from one simple premise: respect and empathy for each other as human beings, each carrying lived experience that can shape how we respond.

That's as true for clinicians as it is for parents. Parents can easily fall into using combative language. I am just as guilty, seeing everything as a fight to be won or lost, and this does not help a culture of collaboration and working together for a common aim.

In a similar vein, by not acknowledging what parents bring to the table – their 24/7 life and lived experience of their child's need – clinicians are not laying the foundations for a collaborative, trusting approach.

It's about standing in each other's shoes. We're all human beings, each bringing a set of skills and knowledge to the table. Caring for a child with complexity should be about working together with mutual respect and understanding, but all too frequently the way we communicate with each other does not support or foster that. Not asking someone their name but just calling them 'Mum' immediately dehumanises the interaction. Not introducing yourself and assuming that the parent must know who you are can create a power-based relationship from the start. Care is not the same as caring.

I remember hanging on every word Daisy's doctors told me, and their throwaway comments had a huge impact.

I relied on Daisy's clinical team to help ensure my daughter got the best quality of life possible. I needed them on my side. I worked hard to help them understand what our world was like. I think in many ways I got lucky because we had some brilliant clinicians who took the time and trouble to get to know me as a person and to understand Daisy's world. They had empathy, and we had a relationship of mutual respect and understanding. It meant that when I turned up on a ward worried about Daisy, there were people who knew that my concerns should be listened to. It took a long time to get to that point – there were many fallings out, and not every doctor or nurse interaction was good – but I persisted because I needed to have a team on my side. It shouldn't be like that, however; good communication, empathy and understanding should be the cornerstone of managing and preventing situations of conflict.

But when things start to escalate, it's vital that parents and clinicians are given space and time to talk through the issues, to even accept that there is an issue and to find a way through it. As I've learned more about the role of mediation, I'm surprised about how little awareness and understanding there is of what it is in a medical context and how it could help. I asked Karina what would have made the difference in her situation and straight away she answered: mediation. She, too, just did not know that this was even a possibility; it was not something that was even mentioned. Fortunately, the tide is turning as more hospitals turn to mediation to provide an independent and safe space to work through disagreements between clinicians and parents, to try to avoid escalations that could end up in court.

Parents need better support to know where to turn and what to expect when things go wrong, not framed as a complaints process but as a 'how to guide'. Parents have no training to prepare them when they find themselves caring for a very sick child. Very quickly, they have to learn a new language and get up to speed with how everything works within the system in order to support and advocate for that child.

I keep thinking about chaplaincy services and whether there's a need for advocacy support for parents who are finding their way around the system which is not framed in religion. A sort of translation and navigation service to help them get up to speed quickly.

Following their son's death, Charlie Gard's parents have focused their attention on developing and gaining support for a new piece of legislation called 'Charlie's Law'.[5] Its aim is to avoid the protracted

---

5 Charlie Gard Foundation (2023) 'The launch of Charlie's Law.' https:// thecharliegardfoundation.org/charlies-law/the-launch-of-charlies-law

legal processes they personally experienced when communication broke down with the team treating their son and to find ways to avoid cases going to court.

This includes providing provision for ethics committees across NHS trusts to consider and discuss difficult and complex cases and, crucially, access to mediation services for families and clinicians to try to work through differences and rebuild trust.

The internet has opened up avenues and access to support and information that have completely changed the nature of how parents can approach the challenge of parenting a child with complex needs. It often means that the parents are better informed than doctors when it comes to their child's condition.

Gene therapy, novel drugs, medical technologies – these all bring hope for improved quality of life and potential cures. All come with an opportunity cost. Resources are ultimately finite.

Parents are attending appointments armed with information and evidence. They are educating clinicians on new treatments and approaches that could benefit their child.

Breakthrough gene editing techniques such as CRISPR[6] have opened up a world of possibility for children diagnosed with a genetic disease. Disease support groups buzz with clinical trial updates. Parents live in hope that a promising new drug will be available in time to treat their child.

How do I feel about that? I really don't know. I counted myself lucky that Daisy was born in a time when geneticists were beginning to understand a lot more about her condition. The parents of the children before her taught us so much. And, in the same way, the clinicians caring for children born after Daisy have learned so much from her.

In 2021, the first child in the UK with a diagnosis of the life-limiting disease spinal muscular atrophy (SMA) received what was described as 'the UK's most expensive drug'. Zolgensma is a

---

6   NewScientist (n.d.) 'CRISPR: A technology that can be used to edit genes.' www.newscientist.com/definition/what-is-crispr

single-dose gene therapy treatment[7] which has the potential to dramatically improve the quality of life of patients diagnosed with this life-limiting and devastating disease.

The price tag is £1.7 million, but if it's given early enough, it has the potential to stop the disease in its tracks, preventing mobility and breathing issues from developing or progressing. Promising early research studies show age-appropriate development for children at 5+ years post-treatment.[8]

If someone had offered us the opportunity for Daisy to be treated with a drug like Zolgensma that targeted Costello syndrome, would I take it? Probably. But let's not forget, Zolgensma may be the world's most expensive drug, it may be the best hope for a parent whose child is diagnosed with SMA, but it's not a cure. The child will still have SMA, but the hope is that their life will be extended as a result of the treatment. The hope is the impact of the disease will not be as severe. But they will still need care and support, and their parents will need to continue to fight to get this care and support.

Not every child is a candidate for the new drug, and for some it's just too late.

Without gene therapy treatment, a baby who is diagnosed with the most severe type of SMA can have a life expectancy of two years. My friend Natalie's son, Louie, was born with the most severe form of SMA. We live within a few miles of each other and met through the hospice.

---

7   NHS England (2021, 8 March) 'NHS England strikes deal on life-saving gene-therapy drug that can help babies with rare genetic disease move and walk.' www.england.nhs.uk/2021/03/nhs-england-strikes-deal-on-life-saving-gene-therapy-drug-that-can-help-babies-with-rare-genetic-disease-move-and-walk

8   Novartis (2021) 'New Zolgensma data demonstrate age-appropriate development when used early, real-world benefit in older children and durability 5+ years post-treatment.' www.novartis.com/news/media-releases/new-zolgensma-data-demonstrate-age-appropriate-development-when-used-early-real-world-benefit-older-children-and-durability-5-years-post-treatment

Natalie's story

I often think of Natalie when I am involved in training or speaking at an event. Probably out of all the stories I've gathered, hers has impacted me the most. Her learning curve was steeper than that of anyone else I've met, and without prior life experience, recourse to mediation or the courts, she was able to achieve a positive result for her son when the odds were against her.

Like many children diagnosed with SMA, Louie seemed to be a healthy baby and hit his initial developmental milestones. A few months after his birth, however, Louie began to show signs that things were not right. His muscle tone seemed to change, and Natalie found herself going back and forth to the GP and then the hospital for various developmental issues that were beginning to emerge with her first child. His symptoms spiralled, and within a short time he was on a ventilator in intensive care diagnosed with SMA with respiratory distress, known as SMARD.

Natalie was told that her son would never be able to breathe independently again. Any independent movement he had gained would be lost, and his condition would continue to deteriorate.

The team caring for Louie met with Natalie and her partner and tried to persuade the couple that it was in Louie's best interests to take him to a hospice and remove his breathing support. To let him die.

'Those meetings were so daunting,' Natalie told me, 'and I really struggled in the hospital. I felt like everyone was against us. I remember one nurse in particular constantly telling me when his oxygen levels desaturated that I'd never be able to bring him home and he would never be stable enough.'

But Natalie refused to accept that removing his breathing support and letting him die was the only option. 'Not knowing if your child will live or not, when you desperately want them to, is like hell on earth. I felt as though I was in limbo,' she told me. 'So I did my research, I spoke to charities and I met other families caring for children with the same condition as Louie.'

Through these conversations, she found a professor who was a specialist in SMA, and he agreed to offer a second opinion. He was able to persuade Louie's doctors that it would be ethically right to perform tracheostomy surgery on her son. Louie did not have brain damage; he had awareness of his world and what was going on around him. Despite the poor prognosis and shortened lifespan, performing a tracheostomy would allow Louie's parents to be trained to undertake his care at home. To be able to have him in their lives for as long as possible.

'I was shocked when Louie's consultant told me that he would be having the tracheostomy surgery,' Natalie said. 'I really thought we would end up going to court, and I'd already spent hours filming Louie and writing notes to prepare.

'When Louie had the tracheostomy, I felt like that this was his second chance at life and I was determined to do everything in my power to make sure he had a good life, including doing all the medical care that was necessary for him to live. I literally would have done anything for him.

'For me, I felt that Louie deserved a chance to live. He was still the same baby, but now he needed a ventilator to help him breathe. At that point, he was still doing all the same things that he could do before he was ventilated, and despite knowing that he would need a tracheostomy and be attached to a ventilator, I did feel that he would have a good life and I was determined that he would have a good life.'

Natalie was fortunate – in fact, I'd go as far as to say lucky. She found another expert, she did her research and she was able to present a compelling case that changed the minds of the treating team. Convinced them that despite the diagnosis and the burden of treatment, Louie could still have a good quality of life. Knowing what I know now, it's shocking that Natalie and her partner were told that it would be in Louie's best interests not to perform a tracheostomy surgery and instead remove ventilation and allow him to die. Louie was developing, he was not cognitively impaired, he was not experiencing pain. He was diagnosed with a degenerative mitochondrial disease, but that was no reason to assume that he would not benefit from tracheostomy surgery and home ventilation.

Thank goodness Natalie did her due diligence and sought out a second opinion. A robust case was put to the team that performing the surgery would be in Louie's best interests. This convinced them to change their minds and agree to performing tracheostomy surgery to maintain Louie's life support rather than removing it. The arguments were sound, the case was clear-cut. The second opinion worked, and the evidence convinced the doctors treating Louie to change their minds.

You can see why parents will seek out second opinions when they hear stories like this. Of course we will. If Natalie had sat back and just accepted what she had been told, her son would have died. But as we can see from all the cases I've shared, every child is different, every scenario is different. That's why value judgements of what is the right thing to do are not appropriate. It requires research, conversations and collaboration in order to come to a shared consensus of what will be the best thing for the child. It's not easy for anyone involved.

I become really frustrated when doctors talk about life expectancy, because how can they know how a child will respond? If caring for a child with a rare and complex disease involves 'academic guesswork', as I was told when Daisy was little, then surely giving some sort of prognosis on how long they will live is just guesswork, too? In fact, the UK SMA parent organisation states that even in the severe form of SMA that Louie was diagnosed with, prognosis depends on each child and the interventions that are put in place.

There is no doubt that the decision to perform a tracheostomy prolonged Louie's life. Natalie was 21 when he was born, and she cared for him 24/7. Within a couple of years of being at home, Louie developed intestinal failure and became TPN dependent. Natalie was then trained to put up his drip and manage all the risks that come with a central line.

On the face of it, you could think that Louie didn't have a great quality of life – ventilated, paralysed and TPN dependent. But his mind was intact, and Natalie and her family tirelessly fundraised and raised awareness of his rare disease in order to buy him the equipment and support that he needed in order to maximise his quality of life. He became a big brother to three younger brothers, and Natalie and her partner created memories with their young family with Louie at the centre.

One day, only a couple of years after Daisy had died, I was out walking when I received a message on my phone: Louie had died. His death was unexpected; he had been in surgery for a minor procedure, but he did not survive.

Louie lived for seven years, well beyond the prognosis he was given. He lived because his parents asked for a second opinion from an expert and that expert was able to present a robust case for why Louie should have a tracheostomy. Who knows, in prolonging his life, maybe one day Louie would have been a candidate for a gene therapy treatment and any further deterioration could have been prevented or reversed.

Collaboration and communication coupled with Natalie's deter-mination to leave no stone unturned in her quest to keep her son alive meant that the best outcome for Louie and his family was achieved, and despite his early and unexpected death, he enjoyed life with his family at home.

What if that hadn't worked? Would Natalie have escalated her campaign? Gone to the press and the media? Resorted to legal action? She was gathering evidence in preparation, filming her son in hospital, convinced that the only resolution would be via the courts. Hindsight is a great thing, but really who knows? As a bereaved mother, it's not something she reflects on; she'd rather focus on the time she got to spend with her son.

She left no stone unturned, and the approach worked. You can't blame her for trying, just as you can't blame all of the other parents for doing the same. But it's how these parents are then supported – with medical evidence and knowledge, working collaboratively with their child's team to come up with the appropriate solution for the child – that is key. And those conversations have to start early. Trust has to be built up immediately.

Can you imagine how Natalie felt hearing from the nurses caring for her son that he would never be stable enough to come home? How must that have felt when all she wanted was to explore every option to find a way to bring him home safely? We parents hang on every word as we try to do the right thing for our child, and those words stay with us.

◇ CHAPTER 21 ◇

Daisy's Death

THE YEAR AFTER ANDY DIED OF CANCER was the toughest of my life. I had no time to even think about what had happened, how I had held my husband's hand as he took his last breath in our bed, in our home. My children needed me.

The day after he died, I went to see Daisy at the hospice. I was so grateful that they had opened up their emergency bed so that she would be cared for at this time. I was barely functioning at that point.

I went into her room and got into bed with her. She knew what I was about to tell her. We had made sure that we did not hide Andy's illness from Daisy. I didn't want to give her any false promises, but I also didn't want to scare her.

As I told her that Daddy had been very poorly and the doctors could not make him better, she used the Makaton sign for 'sad' and said, 'Bye bye, Daddy' – she knew exactly what had happened. She, like all of us, was broken-hearted.

Although Daisy had a learning disability, I knew very well that she was still able to feel worried, anxious and stressed. She was very aware that her health and her physical abilities were deteriorating, and now she was very aware that her daddy had died.

Over the years, I had become very concerned about providing space for all my children to articulate their feelings and be open about what was happening. My older children had benefited from play therapy at the hospice, and over the years each of them had found some form of talking therapy really helpful.

I struggled to find support for Daisy's mental health needs, how-ever. There really was nothing available for children with complex medical needs who also had a learning disability and relied on a combination of some words and simple sign language. I knew that while Daisy's communicative skills were not fluent, her receptive skills definitely were. She knew exactly what was going on, what people were saying and what was happening in her world.

I would be furious with doctors and nurses who talked over her as if she was not there, or who did not engage with her – after all, would they treat another ten-year-old girl the same as they treated my daughter?

I just couldn't find anyone to support Daisy with helping her articulate her thoughts and feelings about what was happening in her world and to her body. Every service seemed to be geared towards children who could speak or who only had a mild learning disability.

That's where Daisy's wonderful school helped. The deputy head, who had known Daisy since she was a little three-year-old in the reception class, made it her mission to find help for her. She knew Daisy well enough to know that this was a child who needed support not just for her physical health but also her mental health. She understood that many of her behaviours, increasingly labelled as 'challenging', were rooted in utter frustration, fear and anger at the loss of her abilities and not being able to communicate how she felt about it.

Eventually, she found a solution, and Ella came into Daisy's life.

As a dance movement psychotherapist (DMP), Ella's role was to create a trusting relationship with Daisy in order to allow her to enter into Daisy's world and help her support her emotional well-being and mental health in a non-verbal and creative way.

As Ella explains in my book *Goodbye Daisy*:[1]

[Daisy] knew what she wanted to say, and it was up to us to find a way into her world to understand what she wanted us to know. In our therapy sessions this communication was through symbolic

---

1   Nimmo, S. (2018) *Goodbye Daisy*. Illustrations by Helen Braid. Hashtag Press.

play and body movement. Our focus was on building a trusting relationship in which Daisy could feel comfortable enough to let me understand what she was feeling, seeing and sensing.

Daisy used her movement therapy sessions to play out (using various props, including medical equipment, music and toys) what she was experiencing in her life. She was able to explore her feelings and how out of control she could feel at times. Her therapy sessions helped her articulate through movement and play how she was managing to live with the continuous challenges she faced at both a physical and emotional level.

I worked with Ella, Daisy's teachers and her speech and language therapist to develop a photo book, which we used to help Daisy and her medical team prepare for any operations, procedures or planned inpatient stays. Using these 'social story' and visual resources helped to give the medical team a deeper understanding of how much Daisy understood and how much she needed to understand. Like so many children with medical complexity, there was so much more going on under the surface.

We fought really hard to ensure that Daisy's DMP sessions were funded as part of her overall support package within her education, health and social care plan (EHCP). We knew how important this support was for Daisy's emotional and mental health. It was a vital outlet to allow her to be a little girl and not just a patient. It was an opportunity for Daisy's voice to be heard, for her to feel listened to.

I firmly believe that every child who is diagnosed with a life-limiting condition should have access to the right psychotherapeutic support to help them articulate their feelings. I fought hard to find support for Daisy and to ensure it was funded regardless of whether she was at school. In a time when support for mental health issues is very much on the agenda, we need to ask how we are supporting children with learning disabilities and their mental and emotional health.

Can you imagine what it must be like to know your body is breaking down, to know that you are getting sicker and sicker, to feel as though anyone is listening to you and valuing your feelings about what is going on in your world?

As we entered 2017, I instinctively knew that this would be my last year with Daisy. I struggled with the thought of coping with this long and painful deterioration. Daisy's chest was getting worse, she was pale and she needed to spend most of her time in bed. It was cruel watching her slowly fade but still be so alive.

Daisy, as always, called the shots.

Parents of children with medical complexity have an almost sixth sense when knowing when something is not right with their child. I knew that what was a normal range for one child was not the same for Daisy. It's really common for such chronically sick children to compensate well. An inexperienced doctor might miss the fact that the child is very poorly if they only compare them with the norm among their peer group. So many parents have told me that it's another reason they need to be heard: living with your child 24/7, you see the subtle changes that indicate something is not right. I knew that Daisy was not well. I didn't know if she was about to become septic or she was anaemic or what was going on, but fortunately when I took her to the A&E department at our local hospital, we were met with our dream team of doctors and nurses.

In the 12 years of Daisy's life, I was never once allowed open access to the children's ward. If she was ill and I suspected she needed hospital care (bearing in mind that I did everything in my power to avoid a hospital admission for her by managing at home), then we had to go via A&E. Fortunately, we were able to skip the waiting room, and thanks to Ruth, Daisy's neonatologist, summary notes were always kept in a file on the unit.

It was hit and miss knowing if the doctor greeting us on arrival would have actually read the notes or have even met Daisy before. That day in January, we were met by Graham, and I breathed a sigh of relief. He had been a registrar while Daisy was a neonate and had a reputation among the parents as one of the good guys – one who listened to the parents, who made the effort to understand our world.

Daisy was admitted, and the nurse in charge on the ward that day was Gina. Again, I knew we were in safe hands; she knew our family well and had frequently seen Daisy at her sickest.

It felt serendipitous. Even Ruth was the attending consultant on the ward that week. All these professionals who knew Daisy well were there. They made things happen, and I did not have to try to explain or justify my feelings of unease about what was happening with my daughter.

As the team made calls to Daisy's specialist hospital and discussed a possible transfer, Ella called me.

It was Daisy's therapy day: would she be up for a session?

'Absolutely!' I replied. I knew deep down that this might be one of her last sessions with Ella.

When Ella arrived, I fiercely protected the session, stopping doctors from seeing Daisy, allowing her this time with her therapist. I pinned up a 'do not disturb' sign on to the bed curtains and allowed Daisy, clearly deteriorating, some space.

Ella wrote about it movingly in *Goodbye Daisy*: 'This was our last session. This time, the session was in real time; the medical team, the medical kit, the hospital sounds, the pain, the curiosity and the courage.'

Daisy was transferred to the gastro ward at Great Ormond Street Hospital. Again, she was greeted by familiar faces – nurses who had known her for many years. Daisy was deteriorating before my eyes. All of the things that we normally did to stabilise her – adding in a new antibiotic, extra fluids, specialist infusions – they were not working.

Daisy was scheduled for a colonoscopy to see what was going on with her intestinal system and whether this was causing the problem. But it was delayed because she was too anaemic and needed a blood transfusion. Daisy had received multiple transfusions in her life, but for the first time ever she developed an adverse reaction to this one. Her heart rate skyrocketed, and the decision was taken to stop mid-transfusion.

Her cardiologist came to review her and found that her heart condition had worsened. Daisy was becoming more and more lethargic, and I knew that this was it. I was witnessing the beginning of the end.

She barely responded when her siblings came to visit. I knew then that things were bad, and my children knew too. They had seen their father die the previous year; they knew that they were about to experience the death of their little sister.

All Daisy wanted was to go home and see her beloved dog, Pluto. I bought her a toy dog and arranged a visit from a therapy dog, but they weren't Pluto. I called a friend and asked her to take him to the groomers to be washed and bring him up the next day, and I would ensure that, by hook or by crook, Daisy could see her dog. Maybe this would give her the lift she needed.

It wasn't to be. Over the evening, Daisy's condition deteriorated. People came and went. Calls were made. I sat in a daze by her side, exhausted and numb, trying to answer the myriad of questions being thrown my way, trying to keep other people updated. I was so grateful to my old school friend Lisa, an A&E consultant who was working a night shift in a hospital in Edinburgh. She was there responding to my texts all night as I asked her questions about what was happening and what various results meant.

A doctor came into Daisy's room at about midnight. She was from the intensive care outreach team, there to assess Daisy and to try to stabilise her. The team worked all night on her, pumping various drugs into her, trying to get fluids in to stabilise her blood pressure. By now, Daisy was on oxygen; her breathing was deteriorating, and she was exhausted and struggling to breathe.

During a small window where things were quiet, I tried to get some sleep in a nearby hotel. I knew how much of a fighter Daisy was. This could go on for days or weeks; it could only be the beginning of the end.

My head had barely hit the pillow when my phone rang. It was the nurse in charge: 'We have decided to transfer Daisy to intensive care.'

As I ran along the dark street back to the hospital, I looked up at the sky and, in my head, I shouted at Andy: 'You can't have her yet!'

I don't believe in God and I don't know what happens after we die, but I'd always told Daisy that her daddy was in the stars in the sky, and at night we would wave to daddy. I knew that her time had come.

The work to stabilise Daisy in the intensive care bed was non-stop. When we arrived on the unit, Daisy was still awake and conscious, but she was clearly so very poorly. I just tried to be my usual cheery self with her, telling her what was happening, trying to reassure her. I helped insert her Mitrofanoff catheter into her bladder as the nursing staff caring for her did not have much experience of that sort of stoma and I didn't want them to cause Daisy any unnecessary pain.

Daisy was strong, she was a fighter, and my spirits were lifted a little as she fought with the nurses as they tried to insert an arterial line in order to monitor her blood pressure. I hated having to hold her down – so many times I had to hold her down as she underwent awful procedures – but I knew that having this line in would help try to find the right combination of drugs to reverse this spiral.

It seemed as if everything was going wrong. I'd seen Daisy poorly before, but she'd bounced back and surprised us. This time, the bounce back was not happening.

The consultant intensivist came to see me. 'There's clearly a lot going on,' she said. 'We've added in extra antibiotics and antifungals. We need to find out which bug is causing this overwhelming infection.'

She continued: 'I think she's now at the stage where we need to help her breathe.'

I could see that coming. I'd seen it before. Daisy was struggling to breathe, and that was making her exhausted, which made every breath even more difficult to take. She could not continue like that. I agreed that she needed to be ventilated now.

'I think we should also involve the palliative care team,' the consultant continued.

I think I actually laughed out loud. Thank goodness the nurse who was with me pointed out that Daisy was well known to the palliative team. Can you imagine if, on her deathbed, that was the first conversation about involving palliative care?

I kissed Daisy goodbye before the doctors got to work to intubate her so that the ventilator could take over her breathing. She was struggling hard to breathe, and as I left the ward to wait for them to finish, I felt a sense of relief. Maybe with the ventilator working for her, she could rest, and we could try to find the cocktail that was needed to reverse this downward spiral we found ourselves in.

When the consultant called me back to Daisy's side, she explained that they wanted to get a sample of the fluid that was filling Daisy's lungs in order to get a better idea of what bugs were overwhelming her body. She was clearly septic and had acute respiratory distress. I immediately agreed. I just wanted to know if there was anything that could be done to pull her back from the brink safely.

I sat in the parents' room while the specialist physiotherapist began the bronchial lavage procedure.

And that was when the crash alarm sounded.

I knew that if Andy had been alive, he too would have agreed with me: this was it, this was the end. We were at the point of no return.

Although the crash team managed to restart Daisy's heart, I knew that whatever happened now, the Daisy I knew and loved, the girl who wanted to be a little girl, play with her dog, go to school, be with her siblings, was no more. The window was now closed.

'There are still options,' the consultant told me. 'We could start dialysis. It may give her a few more days – that might give us time to get on top of the sepsis.'

I knew she had to give me all of the options, but as I looked at the monitors, the racing trace of her heart rhythm, the blood pressure that could not be stabilised, the ventilator working on its highest settings, I knew that it was time to let my little girl go.

'Can I take her home?' I asked. I knew about compassionate extubations. When a child is at end of life, arrangements can be made with the palliative care or hospice nursing team for the breathing support to be removed in the hospice or home setting. I only knew about this because, on a previous occasion when Daisy had been septic and needed a ventilator, it had been mentioned as an option if she deteriorated to the point of no return.

'It's too late, Steph.' Our palliative care nurse was with me now. She had known Daisy for years, first when she was a lead nurse in our hospice and, more recently, when she had joined the hospital palliative team. 'She's just far too unstable now, even to go to the hospice, let alone home. There's a risk she could die in the ambulance on the way.'

There was no way I wanted that for Daisy. I wanted her to have peace, not to feel that, in her last moments, she was being moved and hearing unfamiliar sounds and voices.

I knew that she just needed minimal interference now, to just be surrounded with love and familiar voices.

'Please just keep her alive long enough for her brothers and sister to say goodbye,' I said. 'I need them to see her, to know that we did everything we could.'

In many ways, I hated doing that – watching the nurses just pumping fluid into Daisy to try to maintain her blood pressure, doing whatever they could to keep her going... I didn't want that for her, but I also had to think about her siblings. They had barely begun to process the death of their father; I needed to give them a choice about whether they wanted to be there when their sister died. I needed to give them a chance to see her one last time.

Theo and Xanthe caught a taxi from home. They hadn't gone to school that day; they knew that the end was close. Jules had decided he needed the familiarity of school, and I will always be eternally grateful to the teacher who drove him 40 miles in her car into the centre of London so that he could be with his sister.

We gathered around Daisy's bed. My kids knew that these were their final moments with her. I explained that we were going to remove the breathing tube and let her go. I asked them if they wanted to be there for her final moments.

Jules and Xanthe decided they wanted to just say their goodbyes then and there, and sit in a private room nearby while the tube was removed.

'I want to be there, Mum,' Theo said. 'Dad's not here. You should not be alone.' He was 19.

'We can move Daisy's bed to a private room if you want,' the palliative nurse said, 'to give you all more privacy.'

I said no. I didn't want any more disruption for my girl. Instead, the staff very discreetly moved a neighbouring bed a little further away and pulled the curtains around Daisy's bed. I found out afterwards that everyone on duty on the unit knew what was happening. Noise was kept to a minimum; people kept a respectful silence.

Gradually, lines were removed ready for the final tube to come out.

My only request was not to hear any alarms at the end; I couldn't bear the thought of those sounds signalling the final death knell.

I nodded to the consultant.

'It's time.'

We put Daisy's iPad on the pillow next to her and played her favourite songs. I knew that the last thing to go would be her hearing, that she would be able to hear my voice as she took her last breaths.

The tapes holding the endotracheal tube in place were removed, and the ventilator was switched off.

'Go and dance in the stars with Daddy, my darling girl. I love you to the moon and back,' I told her.

Two breaths. Two short gasps.

A trickle of blood-stained fluid ran out of her mouth.

My beautiful girl had left us. I had to do the most selfless thing I could ever imagine, go against my instincts as her mother and let her go, knowing I would never hear her call me Mummy, feel her arms around my neck as I carried her or bury my head in her mop of curls ever again.

I got into bed with my still-warm 12-year-old daughter and hugged her. A light had gone out in our lives. Our family of six had become a family of five the previous year; now we were a family of four.

Unimaginable.

In the end, it was a good death. Because despite being in hospital, on an intensive care ward, surrounded by machines, I felt we had a choice. I felt that both Daisy and I were in control. I truly believe that she knew it was her time, and because of our opportunity to think about how far we would go, I felt a sense of calm that I had done the right thing.

When I interviewed Rosie, I asked her whether Matthias had known that he was dying. He didn't have a learning disability, and he'd been ill for a relatively short length of time. I had prepared for 12 years for that moment. What was it like for her at the end?

'It was clear that the tumour was now out of control, and the oncologist said that there was no more that could be done – no more chemo, no more active treatment,' Rosie told me.

'Did you know, Steph, we lived around the corner from the hospice and we had no knowledge of its existence until the team told us that Matthias's care was just too full-on for him to come home, and they thought it would be best if he was transferred there for pain management.'

And so the family found themselves at the hospice, with a little boy who was no longer able to eat or drink properly because of the huge tumour growing uncontrollably inside him.

'Mummy,' Matthias said to Rosie when they were settled in. 'If I don't eat or drink, I will die, wont I?'

And Rosie replied, 'Yes, my darling'

'But I'm only ten years old,' he told her.

'And you have given me the best ten years of my life,' his mother responded.

And then they spent an hour talking and making plans: what blanket and toy he wanted with him at the end, what he wanted his brothers to have.

Rosie told me that after that conversation, it was like a weight had been lifted from her shoulders: her child had accepted that he was going to die and was preparing for it.

Catherine's story

Alicia was an important part of Daisy's early years in hospital. Alicia had cystic fibrosis (CF) and was frequently in and out of hospital for antibiotic infusions and treatment. Daisy was the same age as Alicia's little brother, and as the two girls were often in our local hospital ward at the same time, she would always come over to wave to Daisy through the window of the cubicle and draw pictures for her.

'I'd thought that CF was a death sentence when we first had that diagnosis, when Alicia was a baby,' Catherine told me. 'But I learned, in time, that it's not a death sentence, that it can be managed, and with good treatment, Alicia could have a good quality of life and live a long life.'

And for a while, that was the case. But as time went on, Alicia began to need more and more treatment and hospital stays.

The girls were often in Great Ormond Street Hospital at the same time, Daisy on the gastro ward, Alicia on respiratory, and Catherine, Alicia's mum and I would be secretly glad that we were in together so that we could sneak out for an occasional drink at the local pub, just to have some semblance of normality.

It was becoming clear that Alicia's lung function was deteriorating to the point where she was going to need to be listed for a transplant. The family were already now using the same hospice as us for respite, although we all just assumed that one day Alicia would get a new pair of lungs and life would improve, just as we had seen with many other families caring for a child with CF. There was no talk of end-of-life plans; hospice was as much to give Catherine a break as it was for Alicia to have some of her care outside of the hospital setting.

There's lots that can be done to treat children with CF; palliative teams don't really get involved these days, I thought...

But every child is unique, and a diagnosis is not always a predictor of prognosis.

As always, Daisy and Alicia were in Great Ormond Street

Hospital. Daisy was having surgery and her recovery was not going to plan; Alicia was in for a chest infection that was becoming worse.

My phone pinged on the ward one morning. It was Catherine: 'Need to talk, bad news.'

I met her in the coffee shop on the ground floor.

'She's dying, Steph,' Catherine told me.

No transplant. Nothing. Alica's little ten-year-old body was becoming overwhelmed; her lungs were struggling, and she was slowly drowning. Even if she was listed for a priority urgent lung transplant, it was too late: she was too ill.

Catherine was told that there was nothing more that could be done for Alicia, and now it was a case of trying to keep her as comfortable as possible and to make some decisions about her care.

'Alicia knows,' Catherine said. 'She told me this morning that she won't be going home from hospital this time, that she's going to be an angel.'

That's when they were introduced to a palliative consultant, the same one who was already caring for Daisy.

'That consultant made an awful situation and difficult decisions so much easier,' Catherine told me as she recalls that first meeting. 'She was just so kind and open. She helped us see how we could help Alicia through this final stage, how we could be empowered about doing the right thing for her.'

Catherine was very clear that she did not want Alicia ventilated, that it would just prolong the inevitable and put her through too much distress. She just wanted her daughter to be comfortable and out of pain. Alicia was already starting to hallucinate as the build-up of carbon dioxide in her lungs affected her brain. I went over to the respiratory ward just a few days before she died to see her and say my goodbyes. This beautiful little girl with her jet-black hair and big brown eyes was fighting for every breath.

I remember going back to Daisy's bedside and kissing her. Ironically, only a few years later, Catherine was the last non-family member to see Daisy before she died, too; she visited the ward and she, like me, had a sense of death being near. When you live with your child and you see what they can deal with, you also have an innate sense of when it's time – it's how you respond to that sense and whether you fight it or accept it that causes the emotional turmoil that you wouldn't want to wish on any other parent.

Catherine, Rosie, me...we were lucky; we were honoured to be with our child as they took their last breath, to accompany them on their last journey in life. And then, after they died, to have time to adjust, to spend time with our children before accompanying them on their final journey.

CHAPTER 22

Care after Death

I OFTEN THINK OF SARA, Livvy's mum. She put Livvy to bed, seemingly well and stable, and the next day woke up to find her precious child cold and not breathing. Overnight, she had become overwhelmed with an insidious infection and died in her sleep. No chance to whisper any final words, to have one last cuddle or even to make any plans. Livvy was not expected to die, despite a number of brushes with death and her increasing complexity. The family did not have hospice support. They had never had a conversation with a palliative care doctor.

And because Livvy's death was unexpected, and she had not been seen by a doctor recently, the police were involved (exactly the scenario that my friend Saira has put plans in place to avoid).

The time after Daisy died seemed so surreal. There was no weeping or wailing, just utter disbelief. I had prepared for this moment for 12 years. Now she was gone, and it just did not seem real.

The palliative nurse and intensive care liaison nurse stayed by my side, helping me make decisions, making things happen. They showed me a lovely side room that was set aside for bereaved families and asked us if we would like to spend some time with Daisy there. I agreed, and after some careful preparation and shutting of patients' doors, Daisy's bed was wheeled into the room.

We sat there – me, my children, all in their teens – and looked at Daisy. We were numb and exhausted, and it all just had not sunk in.

Nurses came in and asked if I would like them to wash Daisy's body, still in her blood-stained theatre gown. They were so kind and gentle, talking to her as they unpeeled dressings and put gauze over her stoma site. They reappeared with a wooden box.

'We thought you would like this,' one of them said. 'These boxes have been donated by another bereaved family.' Inside was a kit to take handprints and a small wooden box in which to keep a lock of Daisy's hair.

We didn't feel rushed, we were in control, but I instinctively knew what I now needed to do.

'I want to take my baby home,' I told our palliative nurse.

All that Daisy had wanted while she was still conscious was to go home. I'd tried my utmost to get her transferred home to die, but she was too unstable. But I knew that in death there was still a way.

A call was made to our community nurse at the hospice: could she set up a cold mattress on Daisy's bed back at the house, please? I knew I needed to honour Daisy's wishes to come home, and thanks to the wonderful cold mattress, a sort of waterbed filled with coolant fluid and connected to the mains electricity to keep it cold, I was able to do so.

The intensive care liaison nurse called the undertaker. The one thing I did not want was for her body to be taken to the mortuary.

It was going to take a while to sort out paperwork. In the same way that a raft of forms need to be filled in when a baby is born, forms need to be filled in when someone dies. I decided to go home ahead of Daisy with my children; they were exhausted and needed to eat and just be in their own space, away from people, away from the hospital, so that they could process what was happening.

I didn't want to leave Daisy on her own, but the nursing staff reassured me that they would check in on Daisy and make sure she was not left alone for too long. I needed that. It seems crazy – she was dead, this was just her body – but she had been cared for all of her life, and I did not want her to be without someone checking in on her.

Once the undertaker had brought Daisy home and tucked her up in her bed, we closed the front door and retreated into our home. All night, each of us wandered in and out of her room, just looking at her. She looked so peaceful; it really was as though she was asleep.

There were no pumps beeping, no tubes or wires. Daisy looked so tall, stretched out, not constricted by pain and spasms. I tucked her soft blanket around her and surrounded her with all of her favourite toys. I lit a candle and put on a playlist of all of her favourite songs. There was always noise wherever Daisy was; I needed this music to break the silence.

As I sat in the chair in her room, the one that our night nurses would normally sit in during their shift, I felt very peaceful. I'd brought my girl home as I promised. She was no longer a patient; she was a little girl again, tucked up in her bed.

The next day, we needed to make a decision:to keep Daisy at home on the cold mattress until her funeral or to transfer her to her beloved hospice for one last stay.

'She would want to go to the hospice' was the unanimous verdict of my kids. They knew what that place meant to Daisy; it was her happy place, where she could have sleepovers and time away from Mum, just like any other pre-teen girl craved.

So back came the undertaker, and Daisy was safely brought for one final stay at the hospice. The cold room where children normally stayed after they died was already occupied, so the staff set the cold mattress up in one of the spare bedrooms. It was perfect. They had decorated the room and put fairy lights around the bed. Carefully, they helped me dress her in her favourite Disney princess dress, removing the hospital nightgown, the last vestige of her life as a patient. She belonged to us now.

The boys had decided not to come to the hospice; they were happy to stay at home, and I needed them to do whatever was right for them. But Xanthe stayed with me; she needed to spend some more time with her sister. She set to and painted Daisy's nails and applied makeup, delighted that, for the first time ever, Daisy was now still, so she could get it perfect. The final touch was a crown of fresh roses in her hair. It felt ritualistic, dressing Daisy and preparing her, engaging with her death.

'It was so important to me,' Xanthe has since told me. 'I thought I would be scared, if anyone had told me that I would be putting makeup on my dead sister. But I found it so healing. I'm so glad I got to spend that time with her.'

Kevin Toolis has written about how death and dying has become sanitised and almost industrial in his book *My Father's Wake*:[1]

> In the Anglo-Saxon world the very sight of the dead is forbidden, outlawed, pixelated away even on the television. The Irish wake runs with an older wisdom. Rather than denying death, the wake reaches out to embrace the bereaved, the living and the dead in a series of rites.

Engaging with death and Daisy's dead body – the simple rituals of dressing her and putting flowers in her hair – seemed to take me back into a simpler time where the dead and dying were among us, not hidden away, where we did not fear dead bodies. We talk about the dead in hushed tones. And when it comes to the death of a child, it's simply a taboo subject. Western medicine has done so much, after all; how can it still be possible that children die? But they do, and we need to talk about it.

When I interviewed Gemma, she was very clear: 'Children die, Steph; we have to accept it' – and this was from a woman who is not only an experienced palliative nurse but also facing the fact that her own daughter will have a shortened life.

I invited friends to come and visit Daisy, just as they used to visit her when she was in the hospital or staying in the hospice. Most of them had not seen a dead body, let alone the dead body of a child.

'I don't know if I can, but I'll do it for you,' most of them told me. They went into Daisy's room anxious, full of fear at what they were about to face. Their friend's daughter was dead...and yet every single person who came out was happy they had been to see her. 'She just looks so beautiful and peaceful,' they told me. We all cried tears of

---

1   Toolis, K. (2017) *My Father's Wake: How the Irish Teach us to Live, Love and Die.* London: Orion.

happiness; it was tragic and sad, but I gained such comfort from spending time with Daisy, from reclaiming her from the medical world, from just having that calm time together as I readjusted my sails.

Daisy's funeral was held at her school during half-term week. It was beautiful. Xanthe and I had chosen a pink wicker coffin, and it was adorned with pink daisies and roses.

'It takes a village to raise a child like Daisy,' I began my eulogy. And it was so, so true. I looked around the room, and there were people who had been part of Daisy's life at all stages: her school friends, doctors, nurses, carers...many of them spoke at the funeral, and a week later at the memorial that we held in the hospital chapel at Great Ormond Street Hospital. Daisy was part of their lives as much as they were part of hers. A child with a complex condition needs a village, and the entire village felt empty as we mourned for our bright, rainbow girl.

We think about caring for children up to the point of death, but what about afterwards? I was fortunate; I had some knowledge of things like cold mattresses and not having to rush to make decisions. By talking to other bereaved parents beforehand, I'd understood the benefits of taking time before Daisy's funeral and making sure I was involved in her care after death.

In Western culture, death is not part of our everyday lives. We're no longer witnessing it on a regular basis; it's become medicalised, hidden away and not talked about. And because we don't engage so frequently with death, people don't realise that they have a choice – that caring for their child after they have died is as important as caring for them when they were alive. It's the last act of love.

Many faiths have clear guidelines on what should happen after death. In Judaism, for example, it is important to bury the body as soon as possible after death, preferably within 24 hours. In Islam, there are important rituals to prepare the body for burial, including washing at the mosque. Religious customs help guide families and professionals, but where there are no religious laws to adhere to, families and professionals can flounder.

Through conversations with families, it is clear that choices after death are very individualised and vary from family to family. However, what is offered to families is dependent on what is available in each area and also on the understanding and confidence of staff to be able to discuss this.

Once a child dies, the focus of the professionals shifts from caring for the child to caring for the family. There are practicalities that need to happen, but what each family needs and wants can vary.

There doesn't seem to be a clear understanding among medical teams about how to make this switch and to think about how to support and care for a family once a child has died. Some parents may have strong thoughts about what they want to do; others look to the professionals for guidance – feeling disempowered, not knowing what happens next.

Parents need to be able to look back at this transitional time without regret, but if the health professionals don't know what options are available, then families might not realise what's possible.

Sacha's story

Sacha lives every day with the knowledge that she gave her beloved son DD a good death, and with the regret that there were things she wished she had known when it came to the time after death.

'I remember hearing about how you were able to bring Daisy home because of the cold mattress,' she told me, 'and my first thought was that I wish I'd known that; I would have loved to have kept DD home a bit longer, to not have felt so rushed in the time after death. I hated that he went into the undertaker's fridge, and now I know he needn't have.'

Sacha and I met through our work on behalf of the paediatric palliative care charity Together for Short Lives. Like me, she's a passionate advocate for good paediatric palliative care, and our first ever 'in real life' meeting was at the House of Commons at the launch of her new book, *Follow the Child*,[2] on the first anniversary of Daisy's death.

Her eldest son, David, known as DD, had been diagnosed with an aggressive brain tumour, a medulloblastoma, at the age of 11. At diagnosis, the doctors were very optimistic; there was a lot that could be done. Sacha and her husband, Toby, were scared but tried to be positive.

DD was the oldest of three children. Life as the family knew it changed beyond recognition as the couple juggled caring for DD and hospital stays with trying to ensure that their younger children still had a childhood and got to do the 'normal' stuff of playdates and sleepovers.

DD's treatment went on for five years. Family and friends rallied around supporting Sacha and Toby both financially and practically, while the couple supported DD through gruelling surgeries, chemotherapy, radiotherapy and stem cell treatment, always remaining optimistic that they would get through this time and would be able to reclaim some sort of normal life together again.

By the time DD was 16, he was taking his GCSE exams and was predicted top grades. He wanted to go to university, had developed a keen interest in flying birds of prey, was learning about beekeeping and was exploring the Buddhist faith.

He was also showing signs of dementia. It appeared that the years of gruelling treatment were not holding back the cancer in his brain and his cognitive function was deteriorating.

Sacha poignantly describes a car journey with DD where she realised that something was seriously wrong: '[O]n the way back home DD asks me which route we're taking back; I reply and then a minute later he asks exactly the same question. There is nothing in the world like the void of terror, the sickening lurch and impact of pressure that hits the chest when your body responds to an

---

2   Langton-Gilks, S. (2018) *Follow the Child: Planning and Having the Best End-of-Life Care for Your Child.* London: Jessica Kingsley Publishers.

understanding before your brain has even formed a sentence to itself: I knew then.'[3]

The cancer was raging out of control, and Sacha found herself having what she calls 'the difficult conversation' with her son's doctors, the one that she dreaded.

After tests and scans, Sacha, Toby and DD were ushered into the doctor's room. He asked if DD wanted to be there, and Sacha agreed that he should if he wanted to. They had always told him the truth, so that he understood why he was going through the treatment. He was 16 now; he was able to make his own decisions about how much more treatment he wanted to go through.

The oncologist was very direct. 'There's clearly now no chance of curing this cancer,' he said. 'I'm sorry, David.'

'So am I going to die?' DD responded.

The oncologist talked about palliative chemotherapy, but the family were united in their decision.

'We're going home,' said Sacha.

'And please, no steroids,' added DD.

'I promise, only pills to take away pain, my darling,' Sacha told her son. 'And now we're going home to party.'

And party they did – DD was a teenager, after all, and he did not want to be around hospitals anymore. He wanted to have a great big party with all his mates; he wanted fun and laughter.

The family began to make plans. Sacha drew up an advance care plan for DD's end of life. She knew that DD did not want to be in hospital anymore and that he wanted to die at home. The plan captured those wishes and how far the family were prepared to go in terms of treatment and intervention. Sacha found this whole process hugely empowering.

Having DD at home for his final three months involved mobilising a huge amount of medical support: from the local GP services to knowing whom to contact, 24/7, at the hospital, from phone

3   Langton-Gilks, S. (2018) *Follow the Child: Planning and Having the Best End-of-Life Care for Your Child*. London: Jessica Kingsley Publishers.

support from palliative care nurses to the Marie Curie nurses who did night shifts in the last few weeks with DD so that Sacha and Toby could sleep and care for their other children.

There had never been a hospice referral; the focus of the clinical team was always on achieving a cure, and, in fact, it was only after DD died that a specialist paediatric palliative consultant started working at the hospital. Too late for DD, but hopefully not for the children who followed behind. At the very beginning, when DD had just been diagnosed, the family were introduced to a specialist palliative nurse on the oncology team, but Sacha refused to connect with her, believing that somehow she was being told that DD was about to die.

'I didn't understand what palliative care meant, and it was not explained. I had no idea that they're the team that can enable a child to live well, longer, and are involved even for curative treatments where side effects are awful.' How different could it have been for DD, Sacha and the family at the end if those early conversations could have been reframed earlier, so that Sacha could have understood how they could help and engage with them to support her son?

We were fortunate. Palliative care was discussed and the team involved very early on with Daisy. It meant that we were able to plan and discuss her end-of-life care and options. Daisy had taught us so much about these conversations, but when Andy was diagnosed with incurable cancer, our experience was so different. The palliative care team were brought in during the final weeks of his life. It really did feel as though his oncology team were giving up, that palliative care was the final stage rather than a thread that should have run parallel to treatment. Sometimes people recover, sometimes new experimental treatments work – maybe it's better to have palliative professional involvement running concurrently. After all, if the patient doesn't die, the palliative team won't take it personally; they're all about maximising quality of life, not about success and failure.

DD's health deteriorated rapidly; he was having constant

seizures and eventually he slipped into a coma and developed a 'death rattle'. This is the indication that death is near, as the dying person can no longer clear saliva from their throat.

Rosie told me that these are the things she wished she had known when Matthias was dying: what is the process of death, why are all these things happening?

After many long hours, Sacha and her family were woken up by the night nurse so that they could be with DD for his final breath.

'The physical relief of silence after his laboured breathing, which seemed to sum up all of his suffering, was instant. It was like the photo negative of a birth where pain instantly stops and happiness flows.'[4]

After DD died, Sacha felt unanchored and adrift. Her focus had been on achieving a good death for her son; now he was dead, she was grasping around for what to do next.

'We planned for the time before death; there was nothing in place for afterwards,' she told me. And after death is the time when exhaustion hits and you can no longer rely on adrenaline to power you through.

My instinct had been to get into bed with Daisy and hold her straight after she died, savouring every last moment of her warmth and her soft limbs, but Sacha did not want to do that. She didn't want DD's body in the house now that he was no longer alive, but she wanted to take care of his body and wash and dress him herself before his final journey.

Looking back, what Sacha really wanted to do next was to put her dead son in the car and drive him directly to the crematorium herself. She wanted to avoid having to deal with an undertaker. As she told me: 'If only we had been supported by our local hospice, maybe we could have arranged for a cold mattress so that we could have kept him at home until there was a slot in the crem.'

If only someone had thought of this and suggested it to her.

---

4   Langton-Gilks, S. (2018) *Follow the Child: Planning and Having the Best End-of-Life Care for Your Child.* London: Jessica Kingsley Publishers.

When Sacha asked if there was any way she could just take her son to his cremation herself, she was wrongly told that it was illegal to cross county lines (the crematorium was in the next county) with a dead body. She found out later that this was wrong, and it still makes her deeply cross to think about it.

There are so many myths and misnomers about what families can and can't do after their loved one dies. You don't have to deal with an undertaker; you do need to have the relevant documentation in place, but after that the law states that a body must be cremated or buried.

Sacha wanted DD to be cremated as soon as possible. She did, however, want to gather people together in a celebration of his life. This was a huge gathering of friends and family, with music and Buddhist prayers and much laughter.

How we care for a child and their family after death is not something we do well, and if it's done badly, it can leave a lifelong scar. When I was speaking to Sacha, it was clear how much this has affected her. While she is proud that she was able to honour DDs wishes in many ways and was able to care for him in his dying hours at home, not being in control about the events post-death still gnaw at her, years later. She seeks closure in her work to make sure that professionals know what is possible, to know that their work does not end at the last breath of the child.

For Sara, closure came in an unexpected way. Livvy's death was unexpected and, in some ways, unexplained. Sara had walked in to find her precious child cold and lifeless. As with all unexplained deaths, there was a post-mortem and an inquest.

In the time waiting for the inquest results, Sara went through everything over and over: had she done something wrong, had she got Livvy's medications wrong, had she contributed to her daughter's death?

The post-mortem showed that Livvy had died very suddenly of a catastrophic infection that had taken hold of her body, shutting down her organs within a space of hours. There was nothing that Sara could have done differently; it was in part as a result of Livvy's underlying condition, Rett syndrome, and ultimately it was a sad risk that the family lived with. But it was the coroner's words at the inquest that gave Sara comfort.

He reassured her that death, when it came, would have been irreversible, that there was nothing that could have been done and that there was nothing that Sara had done that would have contributed to Livvy's death.

Then he talked about Livvy: how, in examining her in the post-mortem, it was clear how beautiful and loved she was, how her hair was brushed and her nails manicured with polish on them. He talked about Livvy as a loved and precious daughter, a beautiful child. He gave her story a name, and in doing that, he took the trauma and despair that Sara was feeling and framed it around a child who was so loved and cared for and sadly missed.

Before researching this book, I had not really thought about how a coroner's words could provide comfort and reassurance to a grieving family. For Sara, while the coroner would never bring Livvy back, he brought her some closure and peace in his carefully chosen words.

We didn't know how long we would have with Daisy. We thought maybe a year...we got 12 years. After she died, I felt bereft and adrift. The empty wheelchair, a symbol of my loss. But I also felt relief – relief that she was out of pain and that my instincts that Daisy's quality of life had diminished in her final weeks were well founded, but also relief that she would not have to face any sort of future where I would not be there to care for her, where I could not keep her safe. I had lived with the bittersweet dilemma of wanting to keep my child with me for as long as possible but fear that she would transition to adult services and everything that would entail.

CHAPTER 23

Outliving the Prognosis

T HERE WERE TIMES WHEN I WORRIED if Daisy would outlive her prognosis, survive into adulthood. I say 'worried' because what would that mean for her transitioning into adult services? Her care was so complicated; she bounced back from the brink so many times, but she was totally dependent on me for her care and to be her voice.

As she grew older, I felt a huge weight of responsibility to make decisions on her behalf, to try to understand what she would want. If I wasn't around, what would happen to her? Who would care for her, listen to her?

Only a few months before Daisy died, I had a conversation with her intestinal failure consultant. She had suggested that as Daisy had defied the odds over and over, it might be worth beginning very early conversations with the adult intestinal failure team so that they would be prepared to take over her care once she reached 18.

I didn't want Daisy to die, but I didn't want her to live without the care and support she needed to have the quality of life that she wanted. Her care became increasingly complicated with each passing year; at home, I was running the equivalent of a high-dependency unit. If she was admitted to our local hospital, I would often find that the staff there did not have the experience or training to manage many aspects of her care, and this meant that I just could not leave her side.

And beyond the skills needed to set up her IV infusions or

catheterise her Mitrofanoff stoma, Daisy needed someone with her all the time to keep her safe if she had a seizure or needed help – she was not able to use the call button, after all. And outside of an intensive care setting, one-to-one nursing was simply not an option. It's no wonder that most parents of complex children only ever feel completely safe when their child is in ICU. I remember one nurse in the early days telling me to go and get some sleep as Daisy (once stable) was in the care of the best babysitters we would ever have.

Children are outliving their prognosis and surviving into adulthood, but that survival depends on complex care regimens, expensive drugs and specialist equipment.

I worried that Daisy would reach adulthood but knew that she would be dependent on me to advocate for her. After Andy died, I felt a huge burden of responsibility to stay alive and well. This was fuelled by a comment made in passing by our social worker, when she told me that if anything happened to me, she was not sure where Daisy would go as we were struggling to ensure that there were suitably trained nurses available just to take her to school or cover night shifts. There were many gaps when nurses cancelled shifts or those shifts could not be covered, and booking any form of respite was becoming more and more tricky as appropriate levels of staffing could not be guaranteed.

Apparently, if Daisy was staying at our hospice, then they could not take in another child with complex medical needs at the same time. This was the balance that had to constantly be struck. I had to stay alive, but I lived in fear of a time when I might not be able to care for Daisy, to read the subtle signs that told me she was brewing something, to interpret her needs, to just be her voice and advocate.

I didn't want Daisy to die, but I could not imagine a life where she was no longer cared for in paediatric services, where she was classed as an adult, and I was no longer able to make decisions on her behalf. Daisy lacked mental capacity to make decisions for herself; she could clearly articulate her wants and needs on a very basic level, but she would not have had the capacity to agree to a lasting power of attorney arrangement for me to manage her healthcare needs, for example. If Daisy had lived to 18, I would have had to apply to the court of protection to still be allowed to make decisions on her behalf, and that involves lots of long and complicated forms and can take months.

I still live with a mixture of relief and utter sadness that Daisy died at the age of 12. Relief that I was able to give her a good death, to be with her at the end, to be there for her when she needed me, but utter sadness of how everything in our lives had unravelled. I see other children with Costello syndrome doing well, able to read, able to walk, able to make choices, but Daisy's case was extreme; that was never going to happen. I did not want her to endure any more pain or deterioration. I'm sad that she's not here, but I would not want her to suffer any more than she already had. Her window, as we described it to the palliative team, had closed.

But what happens when a young person does have mental capacity? When they can make decisions for themselves, when they outlive their prognosis?

Gillick competence is used in English and Welsh medical law to decide whether a child (under 16 years of age) is able to consent to their own medical treatment, without the need for parental permission or knowledge. Victoria Gillick challenged Department of Health guidance which enabled doctors to provide contraceptive advice and treatment to girls under 16 without their parents knowing. In 1983, the judgement from this case laid out criteria for establishing whether a child under 16 has the capacity to provide consent to treatment – the so-called 'Gillick test'.

It was determined that children under 16 can consent if they have sufficient understanding and intelligence to fully understand what is involved in a proposed treatment, including its purpose, nature, likely effects and risks, chances of success and the availability of other options.[1]

I have often wondered if Daisy would have agreed to the

---

1   Care Quality Commission (2022, 23 December) 'GP mythbuster 8: Gillick competency and Fraser guidelines.' www.cqc.org.uk/guidance-providers/gps/gp-mythbusters/gp-mythbuster-8-gillick-competency-fraser-guidelines

decisions I made on her behalf if she had the mental capacity; would she have looked back and said, 'I'm glad you did that for me, Mum'?

As I was researching this whole area, I came across the story of a young man called Danny Bond. Danny had been born with a rare disease causing complete intestinal failure; he too was TPN dependent for all his nutrition, experiencing the risks and side effects of that method of nutrition throughout his childhood. Danny had the mental capacity to make his own decisions, however, and he was very clear that he did not want to live like this.

He started talking about wanting to die when he was only 13. He had already spent most of his childhood in and out of hospital, becoming increasingly isolated from his peer group; he endured countless surgeries and procedures, and as he grew older, the pain he was experiencing became worse and worse.

Danny made it very clear to his parents that he did not want to live like this any longer and was apparently very rational in his thinking and actions. One day, Danny's mum walked into his room to find he had tried to kill himself. Her instinct took over, and she resuscitated him. He survived. For Danny, it was the worst thing she could have done. He no longer wanted to live his life in this way; the surgeries, infections and pain were just all too much, and in his mind, there didn't seem to be a way out of it. It was the early 2000s, the early days of small bowel and stomach transplants that might have been an option for Danny; paediatric palliative care services were in their infancy, and this also meant that effective pain management and treatment regimens were not immediately available.

Danny attempted to take his life three times. Just after his 21st birthday, he was rushed into hospital with an infection, and his condition rapidly deteriorated. Now that he was an adult, he was able to refuse any more intervention, but he wanted to die quickly, so he decided to refuse any more TPN and starve himself to death. The doctors tried to persuade him that there was more that could be done; funds had been raised for him to go to a specialist intestinal failure hospital in Cincinnati, USA, but Danny had had enough, and he asked his parents to stay by his side to make sure that he could have his wish to die in peace.

The way Danny died had a profound effect on the whole family, but particularly on his mother. 'If I knew then what I know now, I would have chosen for him to be left alone, because all we did was sentence someone to 21 years of hell,' she commented at the time.[2]

Danny's story is bound up with so many complex, ethical issues: the burden of responsibility on parents who have to make life-and-death decisions for their child, the views of the child on their care and even the question of assisted suicide. Everything I know about Danny's case is gleaned from press reports and tracking down a TV producer who was involved with a documentary about his life; this all happened 20 years ago now. I would like to think that some progress has been made, that Danny would not have had to endure the physical and mental agony that drove him to the point that he would rather die than live his life.

Babies, children, young people – they are outliving prognoses, thanks to scientific progress and an increased understanding of symptom care, but there is a price to be paid. What sort of mental turmoil was Danny going through to want to take his own life? And how were his parents supported? As a mother, it's the hardest thing in the world to watch your child suffer; how must Danny's mother have felt as he told her to let him die?

It's no wonder that recent research[3] has found higher incidence rates of common and serious physical and mental health problems and death in mothers of children with a life-limiting condition.

It was only after Daisy died that I was able to really reflect on what I'd been through with her, what I'd witnessed. I was diagnosed with PTSD and underwent two years of therapy. I'm not sure if I'll ever be out of the woods – it's something you learn to live with. The

---

2   BBC Press Office (2002) 'Life etc – parents reveal their anguish at not being able to help their son to die.' www.bbc.co.uk/pressoffice/pressreleases/stories/2002/03_march/08/dannybond.shtml

3   Fraser, L.K., Murtagh, F.E., Aldridge, J., Sheldon, T., Gilbody, S. and Hewitt, C. (2021) 'Health of mothers of children with a life-limiting condition: A comparative cohort study.' *Archives of Disease in Childhood 106*, 10, 987–993.

flashbacks still happen and the moments of 'what if?'; no doubt, all these years later, Danny's mum still feels it, too.

Lucy's story

I met Lucy many years ago when I was invited to speak at a charity event for the children's palliative care charity Together for Short Lives. We had followed each other's blogs, and it was wonderful to meet her in person at long last. We remain firm friends.

Although Lucy had been poorly when she was born and lived her early years with a range of health issues, nothing she was going through would indicate the dramatic downturn in her health that would render her dependent on a wheelchair and TPN by her teens. Prior to that time, she was like any other average little girl – mad keen on horses, spending all of her spare time at the local stables, busy with school and getting on with life. At the age of 14, things started to go very wrong for Lucy. The minor health issues she had experienced became significant and more complex, and she began to rapidly lose weight, unable to eat without vomiting or experiencing extreme pain. She ended up in hospital, and after every avenue was tried, she was started on TPN as she was clearly desperately unwell and in need of nutrition to survive.

Lucy was diagnosed with complete intestinal failure and a multitude of other issues, all stemming from a very rare condition, probably mitochondrial in origin. From being an active teenager, riding and swimming and attending school, Lucy became TPN dependent, unable to walk and unable to manage any of her care needs.

She was told that it was likely that she would not live to see her 18th birthday and was referred to a local children's hospice for support.

But Lucy, like Daisy, defied the odds, despite multiple episodes of sepsis and a constant deterioration in her health. When I interviewed her for this book, she was a few months short of her 28th birthday.

In the early years of her deterioration, Lucy's mum, Kate, cared for her and made decisions on her behalf about her care. Kate still manages much of Lucy's medical care, but now Lucy is in the driving seat about what she wants for her life, about how she wants to live her life.

As Lucy says: 'Remember when you were a teenager, and you had your plans, your goals, your dreams for your life; imagine having all of that taken away from you and being told you were going to die. That happened to me, and it was a turning point in my life.'

I often think about that quote from the film *The Shawshank Redemption* when I think about Lucy: 'I guess it comes down to a simple choice, really. Get busy living or get busy dying.'[4]

Lucy, knowing her time is finite, has got busy living. Despite constant pain and her body failing her, she has been determined to make her mark and to make a difference.

Lucy was awarded an MBE for her work in advocating for people with disabilities and is a recipient of an honorary master's degree from the Open University, but the proudest day for her is the day she came off disability benefits and set up her own business as a disability advocate, public speaker and trainer.

Every day for Lucy is a gift, but it comes at a cost. While she is busy supporting other families in securing care packages and support for their children, she is still fighting for the support she needs. Our social care system is simply not used to supporting young people with the same complexity as Lucy, and yet more and more young people are outliving their prognosis and surviving into adulthood.

'It takes its toll,' she told me. 'I'm advocating for my own needs, fighting to ensure that I get the pain medication I need, but often doctors just don't understand what I need to be able to get through the day and function.'

Lucy is being worn down by the fighting the constant battle to ensure her hard-earned care package is not taken away, to ensure her home is fit for purpose, to just get the pain meds she needs. She, like Danny Bond, is very clear about what she wants for her

---

4   www.youtube.com/watch?v=B1KsZo_foYE

life, and in many ways, like Danny, our system is not geared up to support her wishes.

Lucy's mother still manages a lot of her care; it's not what Kate expected to be doing now that her daughter is a young woman. Every day, she still puts up the TPN infusion, she still opens the door to the night nurses who come to sit with Lucy. They are both living a life a million miles from the one that they had imagined. A few years ago, Kate became very ill and was found to have a brain tumour. One evening, she had a seizure in Lucy's room, and Lucy, unable to move from her bed to help her mother, felt powerless. Kate is in remission following successful surgery, but she still lives with the side effects of her own illness, side effects that she has to ignore in order to support her adult daughter.

I remember the thoughts I had all those years ago, when Daisy was in the neonatal unit: this was it – for the rest of my life, my child would be my child, dependent on me, forever. We do it for love, the care we give our child; we put our own health needs on the backburner, make sacrifices and think little of the impact on ourselves. I know Kate would not change a thing, but how much and for how long can we keep leaning on parents to always be there to fill in the cracks in our broken social care system?

When I was writing this book, I received news that another young woman I have known for many years had died. Amy also had intestinal failure. I'd met her mum, Helen, while we were both staying on the gastro ward at Great Ormond Street Hospital. Amy also had a lot of life to live. She'd received a multi-organ transplant, but a year later the new organs failed and were removed, and Amy returned to life on TPN. I visited Amy at the hospice only a few weeks before she died. She was a young woman full of life and hope; she didn't want to die, she wanted to live – there was so much she wanted to do with her time. She had also outlived her prognosis over and over; medical science had given her many years beyond her original prognosis. Life can be unbearably cruel, yet Amy did not regret a single decision her parents had made for her and she had then made for herself. She just wanted more time.

Daisy had hopes and dreams. In her mix of limited words and sign language, she would tell me that when she was a big girl, she wanted to work with her friends, Singing Hands, a Makaton singing and signing duo; she wanted to help them by handing out stickers to the children who had done good signing at the end of each concert. Daisy had a learning disability, but her life, in its own way, had value.

It's bittersweet. Lucy is empowered and confident; she has made things work for her, and she is making every moment of her life matter. As she says, it's not always doom and gloom; great care and support has allowed her to get to this point. She has grown into a confident, articulate young woman, and her only frustration is that her body is letting her down. Daisy was like Lucy, despite her learning disability. Daisy was clear about what she wanted, how she wanted to live.

Doctors don't know what the future holds for their patients, how they will respond to treatment, how long they will live for. What works for one person might not work for another. It goes back to that academic guesswork question again. Doctors can't predict what the future holds. We really need to stop discussing prognoses and instead think about quality of life and what that means for each individual.

Lucy is alive because of brilliant palliative care support to manage her symptoms. She accepts she is in decline, that every day is a gift. Her team have had to adapt and learn; they are, after all, more used to patients who are at end of life. But working with her team, Lucy has been able to decide what she wants for her life and, when the time comes, for the end of her life.

Daisy would now be 18, and her transition to adult services would have been finalised.. Would they be prepared to fund her expensive medications, her complex care package? Would I still have the energy to speak on her behalf, to advocate for her to ensure that she could live a full but shortened life as an adult? I remain grateful that this is a scenario that I didn't have to face. It could have been so different. I have freedom and my health because Daisy died...and yet I carry the scars and pain with me every single day.

CHAPTER 24

Professionals Are Human, Too

W HEN YOU FIND YOURSELF CARING FOR A CHILD with complexity, you get to meet a lot of medical professionals in all sorts of situations – the community nurses who come to the house to help with dressing changes, paediatricians at the local hospital, specialist consultants at a different hospital, nurse specialists, home nurses and carers, school nurses, community paediatricians, hospice staff...

Every one of them sees a part of our lives. Sometimes it's a curated part. Sometimes we welcome them into our homes, and they see our lives on full display. Some become friends; some are people we don't really gel with but we know that their specialist skills are essential to our child's well-being.

I found that the more specialist the doctor, the further away they were from understanding our lived experience. I soon realised that not all doctors are the same. The friendly team at our local hospital who saw us regularly and got to know my whole family during frequent stays had a different understanding of our world and the impact of caring for Daisy's complexity compared to the specialist consultants at our tertiary hospital. They just saw a snapshot of our world.

Daisy's brilliant and clever neurology consultant was skilled in understanding the various types of epilepsy that Daisy manifested, prescribing the meds that might help, reading the EEG reports that plotted what was going on in her head when she was having a seizure, but did he know what it was like to live every day with a child with complex multi-focal epilepsy like Daisy?

It was after a few clashes with specialists and frustration that they didn't understand my world that I made it my goal to work on helping them understand it. I talked about the impact of what was going on at home and what Daisy needed. I tried to find ways to engage with the specialists. I would have pictures of Daisy at home up on the wall when she was an inpatient, and bring pictures of her to meetings, talk about her world.

Hilariously, Daisy would also frequently contribute. She won over the clever neurology consultant by announcing he could 'Go home now!' whenever he came into her room during an inpatient stay. He had no choice; he had to engage with Daisy and her world. Her gastroenterology consultant soon learned that Daisy associated visits to her clinic with a trip to the shops afterwards as Daisy would announce (with her combination of sign language and limited vocabulary), 'Finish now, shops please.'

It didn't always work, but I needed everyone that met Daisy to see her as a little girl, not just a patient or a diagnosis. It wasn't about fixing her; it was about enhancing and optimising her quality of life. Seeing beyond the individual bits that were broken to the little girl who just wanted to be at home, or school, with her family and friends and her dog.

Just like parents, professionals are human, too, and that means that just like us they come in all shapes and sizes. Some just get it, and some have a hard time engaging and empathising. I think the worst example I ever experienced was an orthopaedic consultant who was assessing Daisy for surgery to lengthen her Achilles tendons and loosen the contractures that were causing her to walk on tiptoe. 'Do you think there's any point?' he asked me 'She's going to die young; is there any point in doing this surgery?'

Orthopaedic surgeons have a bit of a reputation among medical professionals for not having the best bedside manner, but this took the biscuit. Yes, there was a point, because the longer we could keep Daisy mobile and moving, the longer she would have before losing her independence. Being able to stand on flat feet rather than tiptoe would mean she could still participate in things she loved – it was about her quality of life. I like to hope that his concern was about putting her through a surgery and having to wear casts on both legs for a few weeks afterwards, but I'm not sure – it didn't seem to come from a place of concern about Daisy's well-being, in my mind.

I always knew our health services were deeply hierarchical. It concerns me that the people closest to patients – the community teams, the palliative doctors, the primary care doctors – seem to be the ones whose voices are not the strongest when it comes to decisions about patient care. Odd when the aim is to put the patient at the centre and involve patients in co-production of services.

I was recently involved in analysing some qualitative research with doctors, looking at issues around caring for children with medical complexity.[1] We sent a questionnaire to clinicians at all levels and functions, from tertiary hospital specialists to general practitioners. The overwhelming feedback was that there needs to be more joined-up communication between professionals at all levels so that decisions that are made at tertiary level can be implemented back in the community, and for specialist consultants to have a better understanding of the impact of the decisions they make on the day-to-day life of their patients.

Our research showed that the clinicians we contacted want more joined-up communication in order to be able to support families caring for children with complex needs. This sounds great. Sadly, though, there's a huge amount to be done before this can happen. And I'm not just talking about communication between hospitals (over and over, our local team were not kept in the loop about plans for Daisy developed by her specialist team in the tertiary centre). It's also within hospitals, between specialities, between the different professions.

I guess I shouldn't have been surprised when speaking to a

---

1   This was a project for The CoLab Partnership (www.colabpartnership.org.uk).

palliative care consultant recently about her own colleague's understanding of her role and what she did.

'A consultant from another speciality joked to me that I must be good at arranging chairs and handing out tissues,' she told me. In other words, there was no understanding of the value and difference that palliative care support made to the lives of children and their families.

I hadn't realised that. If their own colleagues are not valuing their input, what hope do we have of truly embedding palliative care across all of paediatrics? Of ensuring that every clinician understands that they have a role to play in understanding the whole world of the child, not just the bit they are trying to fix? Or that sometimes children are not fixable but that doesn't mean that they (the clinicians) have failed by involving palliative care?

In conversations with professionals, I have been struck by how different team members may experience different emotions. For example, the sense of responsibility felt by a lead consultant in terms of life-and-death decision making must be huge, or the moral distress of nurses spending hours at the bedside of a very sick child.

I'm guessing that few people enter into medicine or nursing with the specific aim of working in palliative care, so how can these clinicians be supported and trained to know how they can make a difference to families and go home each day with a sense of pride? Maybe this can be achieved, in part, by reframing the way we look at things?

After all, doctors and nurses are supposed to make things better, not allow children to die. But it takes a mind shift to see that it's part of the role. That caring for the dying and not being able to have all the answers are part and parcel of the job of all medical professionals, doctors and nurses alike.

Just as medical professionals should be proud when they have helped cure a child, the work they do in helping a family of a dying child should not be framed as failing in their vocation.

Children die. It's not normal for children to die before their parents in terms of what we expect in the natural order of things, but, unfortunately, it is normal for children to die – children have always died. If we're scared of talking about and engaging in conversations around death as a society, then the death of a child before they reach adulthood must be the biggest taboo.

Fewer children die now, so we're less used to seeing death all around us; we've become immune to it, always expecting that there will be an answer, a therapy and drug. But sometimes there are no answers and we are shocked. Just as families have to live with uncertainty, professionals need to find a way to also admit they don't know and be able to be OK with that.

That's why so many parents have told me that it's actually very liberating to hear a clinician say, 'I don't know.' I haven't come across one parent who felt that those words were a sign of failure. Far from it. And as parents and professionals, we should stop trying to second-guess what is going to happen. Can we really know how long a child will live? How will they respond to treatment? What is around the corner in terms of new therapies?

We don't know; it really is academic guesswork, so why is involving a speciality that can help support symptoms and is focused on maximising quality of life seen as such a negative step? Palliative care teams don't see it as a failure if a child in their care survives beyond their prognosis, but in caring for them, they will have focused on optimising their quality of life and managing their symptoms.

It's about reframing it as professionals: being sad, but acknowledging that not every child that professionals care for will get better and that giving them good care in death is not failing them.

If we are to normalise death and recognise that children do die, then professionals need to take a lead in doing that. They should come into practice with the expectation that their role will include end-of-life care, and this means that, in the majority of cases, the death of a patient should not be treated as an extraordinary event.

As Gemma, the hospice nurse who became a mother to a child with a life-limiting condition herself, told me in Chapter 4, 'I was very aware through my work as a paediatric nurse that children die, and that my child could, and I accepted that very quickly.' If we are to accept that sometimes children are not going to get better, then the starting point has to come from within the system, for all the professionals to support each other, not to see palliative care as a last resort, to understand that not being able to cure a child and have all the answers is not failing and to see enabling a good death as a job well done.

How do nurses, particularly those involved in palliative care, approach new families for the first time? What are their communication strategies?

The hospice nurse told me:

It's about finding ways to build trust. I think it's always intimidating when you meet a parent of such a complex care child because there's inevitably stuff that you don't know about. Practical stuff that you don't know about... Daisy's Mitrofanoff stoma is a prime example – you were always going to be the expert on how to care for that.

As a nurse, you feel like you're letting the parent down at the outset by saying, I'm really happy to look after your child. I don't know how to do that element of care.

By the time I met Daisy, I'd been working in community nursing for many years, but I knew I would never fully know what it feels like to live your life 24/7. We only see a snapshot, and we have to build trust with parents quickly so that they are confident that we can look after their child.

It can feel really intimidating, and you know some parents have had bad experiences, where mistakes were made previously, so they're on their guard, assessing you.

She's right. We're keeping our child alive, we know the intricacies of their care, we live this life full on. And a mistake can be fatal. I would lie in bed awake after stumbling into Daisy's room, blurry-eyed, to administer pain relief, worrying if I'd made a mistake with the dosage. I've spoken to many parents who feel the same; the huge responsibility of keeping our child alive weighs heavy. Not for us the luxury of a second member of staff to check we are administering the correct dosage of a controlled drug; just a hope that we get it right, day in, day out.

That's the dynamic professionals who come into our homes and our lives are entering, and they have to learn to tread carefully.

All the healthcare professionals I spoke to confirmed that they learned to adapt their behaviour depending on what stage of their journey a family was at. If they are caring for a child at end of life whom they've only just met, they will defer to the parents, get on with the job and be a professional presence in the background. It's very different when they care for a child for many years and trust is built up through experience.

Nurses have described the importance of adapting their interpersonal skills to facilitate the building of trust, especially when many families can be so mistrustful of palliative care.

As one of them told me, 'You might be meeting a family for the first time, and they are immediately mistrustful of why palliative care have become involved. I need to find a way of building up that trust so that I can reassure them and we can work together.'

How had these nurses developed the communication skills necessary to build this trust? Their responses were the same. 'Through experience,' they told me. Learning from observing good practice as well as bad practice and doing the job.

There's no training for it. This was confirmed by all the professionals I spoke to for this book. Some had vague memories of one lecture or course on 'communication skills' but nothing really to prepare them for how to work with and talk to parents caring for medically complex children day in, day out. They learn on the job, sometimes from great role models, sometimes from bad examples.

I spoke to a nurse recently who told me that she could see how parents can feel vulnerable and protective of their child, their space and their experience. 'One of my own kids was in hospital recently,' she recounted, 'and there I was in my pyjamas, after a sleepless night next to my child, and the consultant appeared to talk to me, and I realised, this is what it's like for parents like you...'

I remember that feeling well. Months and months of my life sleeping on a plastic-covered mattress next to Daisy, no privacy, feeling quite dehumanised, but expected to then articulate my feelings and concerns calmly to the doctors on the ward round when I was sleep deprived and worried and fed up.

No wonder we use combative language in describing our lives. I used to say that prisoners had more rights than me when we did long stints in hospital. I would go for days without seeing any natural light, existing off microwave meals and coffee.

Every professional only gets a snapshot of the life of a child with medical complexity, and some of them are better at recognising that than others. When I spoke to a friend who is a paediatrician and clinical academic, she told me something that really resonated: '85 per cent of a diagnosis is in the history.'

This is about understanding what has been happening to get to this point where the child is in front of you.

Spending the time and talking to the parents and the child will really help build a picture. I think back to so many of the parents I interviewed for this book who just knew something wasn't right with their child and boomeranged back and forth to hospital just to be sent away until eventually a diagnosis was made. How much time could have been saved, suffering alleviated, if time had been taken to talk and understand the subtleties and nuances that keep driving parents back?

Often, after years of explaining the background, parents carry around a summary of their child's history. Sometimes this is even kept in the child's notes. There's no guarantee that doctors will take the time to read it, though. A top tip I was given about putting anything in writing for doctors to read was to keep it brief – they have a short attention span!

Perhaps that was true of the doctor assessing Daisy in A&E one evening. I was an experienced special needs parent by then, and Daisy had a long and complicated history, a summary of which was kept in the A&E department in anticipation of her regular visits.

'Hi, I'm the doctor on duty tonight. Would you like to go through Daisy's history with me?' he said very jovially

'It's summarised in her notes,' I responded.

'I don't have time to read that, so why don't you just tell me?' he replied.

Head, meet brick wall. I only took Daisy to A&E when I absolutely needed to, and this occasion was following many sleepless nights and days of hoping to avoid hospital. I was exhausted. I didn't have time for this; it was why I'd written a summary for doctors to read so they could hit the ground running.

I know it's daunting, meeting parents like us for the first time. I asked a friend who happens to be a paediatrician about this. How did she feel when she knew she was going to meet with an experienced family caring for a child with medical complexity?

As she replied, I could see the physical and emotional response to my question as she was talking to me...

She took a deep breath and told me that the question I'd just asked her had made her automatically feel a little bit afraid.

'Because it's making me put myself in that situation,' she told me. She continued:

When you meet a family, the child with complex needs and their parents – a family who are living with this whether for a long period of time or if their child is still very small – it's really quite terrifying, as a doctor, going into that situation... You know that not only are the parents going to be strong advocates for their child – so you're already wondering, 'What do they want from me and will I be able to do the things they want for their child?' – but there's also an anxiety around the fact that they are the specialists in their child and what they need, and they will be prepared to fight for what they think is the right thing, and our views on that may differ...

I really appreciated that insight and honesty in response to my question, because it showed the humanity behind the role. Being human, being open, taking off the metaphorical white coat and stepping into the world of the family and feeling what it's like to be them.

The hospice nurses, palliative doctors, community nurses and homecare nurses – they were the ones who really saw our life from all angles (or nearly all angles). As a palliative consultant told me, you can see the difference once you go into a family home:

> In the hospital, there's a certain protocol – it's a formal appointment or conversation, and the parents are coming into our world. When you go to their home, you step into their lives, and then the guard is down. You get to see the piles of washing that they are dealing with, or the fact that the house is super-tidy because that's the only thing they have control over, or the fact that there are other children all competing for attention, the lack of money or resources – so many things that tell you how the family is coping, the realities of life caring for a medically complex child.

We have moved from the biomedical model of medicine to an approach which recognises that patients have a unique experience of the social, psychological and behavioural effects of their disease. In paediatrics, there's another layer – the parent/carer's experience and the role they play in supporting and advocating for their child, often at great sacrifice to their own needs.

Choosing a career in medicine, in whatever field, means choosing a profession that involves working with people and, in the case of paediatrics, working with children and their parents. It's a people thing, and while, as a healthcare professional, you may have gained A* qualifications and be fantastic at drug calculations or some specialist surgical technique, it means nothing if you can't empathise and understand the impact on your patient and their family. On their lived experience and their world.

When Sarah Barclay runs a training session on how to manage conflict in healthcare settings, she starts by sharing a short film that was made by Cleveland Hospital in the USA. It's called 'Empathy – The Human Connection to Patient Care',[2] and it takes the viewer

---

2   Cleveland Clinic (n.d.) 'Empathy: The Human Connection to Patient Care.' https://youtu.be/cDDWvj_q-o8

through a typical day in the hospital with people coming and going, but there's a window into the thoughts each person is carrying in their head, whether patient or clinician. From the doctor who has just learned he's going to be a father to the nurse who is at the end of a stressful 12-hour shift to the daughter coming to visit her dying father:

> Patient care is more than just healing – it's building a connection that encompasses mind, body and soul. If you could stand in someone else's shoes...hear what they hear. See what they see. Feel what they feel. Would you treat them differently?

There is no doubt that the professionals who get it right, who are prepared to walk alongside us and support us on our journey with our child, give a lot of themselves to us, whether they intend to or not.

When I observed the inquest hearing into the death of Karina's daughter Melody, I was floored momentarily when the first witness appeared. It was Daisy's palliative consultant. It really brought it home to me. Here was the consultant who cried when she arrived on the ward just after Daisy died, who read a poem at her memorial service, who had helped us so diligently with our fight for respite – of course, Daisy wasn't her only patient. She had an entire caseload of patients and their families that she was giving her time to.

Over the years, I had become close to many doctors and nurses, mainly those who were the most involved in our lives, at the local hospital, the palliative nurses, hospice teams, community teams... Just as they got to know our family, we got to know them as people, beyond the job title.

It's a difficult one for both sides, keeping boundaries, keeping it professional while also building up a personal relationship in order to build trust. Humanising the interaction is a two-way street. If I'm going to let you into my world, let me into yours a little. Let's call each other by our first names; just let the guard down enough to let me know you're human while also protecting your own privacy.

As Daisy's hospice nurse, told me:

> I think sometimes you just have to let your boundaries drop a little

in order to build a relationship and trust. I don't know what it's like to have a child with complex needs, but I need you to trust that I know what I'm doing. You want to know about the nurse who is looking after your child, so it's a balance between giving a little of yourself without giving too much.

And, of course, this is not just with one family; it's with multiple families and the demands of the job, as my paediatrician friend confirmed:

> It's difficult, standing in somebody's shoes and being compassionate, while also trying to work towards the best thing for the child. It takes time and effort, and all this needs to be balanced with your other clinical duties... And in order to be a good doctor, you have to give a bit of yourself to your job.

Healthcare professionals are certainly not in their role for any financial gain; they do it because they choose to. And often in giving of themselves, they can end up burned out and jaded. Sometimes parents forget this: in the rhetoric of 'them and us', 'they' are humans, too, with their own lives and worries and concerns. And they all have their way of managing the stress of the job because they do become attached to our children, and care about what happens to them, even if there is conflict with the parents.

What happens to our child really does matter to them. So the screaming headlines in high-profile cases, which reduce the people to just cogs in a system, hurt, because the staff caring for the child at the centre of it all have no voice to respond, to say, 'I felt sad too when that child died.'

It was so important to me to involve the nurses, carers, doctors and professionals in Daisy's funeral and memorial. They were grieving, too. They loved my little girl; it was a different love, but her death had a profound impact on them.

As the wonderful agency nurse who took Daisy to school, joined us on days out, spent more time with my family than her own, said at Daisy's funeral:

When I first began working with Daisy I wasn't expecting to meet this determined and strong-willed little girl. I'd read her notes, but a few pages in a folder don't give you the whole story. She let me into her life and became part of my life. I was there to be her nurse, but I got to know her as a little girl, and she stole a piece of my heart.

CHAPTER 25

Conclusion

N IGEL, THE RETIRED HOSPITAL CHAPLAIN I interviewed, told me an anecdote during our conversation which really resonated.

He was describing his first day in the role, as the new chaplain for a hospital trust in the north-east of England:

> It was mind-blowing really. Here I was in this huge hospital, a newbie, with a steep learning curve ahead. A senior colleague came up to me and told me, 'Remember this feeling, because very quickly you'll become part of this organisation. You might not believe it now, but you'll get used to the sights, the sounds, the jargon. Remember this, because how you feel today, on day one of your new job, is how patients and families feel every time they are in hospital.'

That's what it's like for parents caring for medically complex children. We find ourselves parachuted into an alien world, totally out of our comfort zone, forced to take on extreme parenting challenges every day. Who guides us? Who helps us? It's all too easy for health professionals to slip into jargon, to assume that everyone else knows how the system works.

I look back to those early months after Daisy was born. I did not have a clue how hospitals worked. That the nurse looking after your child today won't necessarily be the one looking after them tomorrow. The hospital lingo, the routines, the hierarchies, the job titles and roles. Looking back, I have a sense of how a refugee must feel coming to this country, trying to fit into a new and strange culture.

There is a spirit of self-reliance among parents who find themselves navigating this new and alien world. No one else will sort it for you, so you have to adapt and adjust quickly. There are no guides or teachers to leap in and take control. There are no interpreters; there is no handbook of extreme parenting. Just the dawning realisation that your child needs you to get your head around it all because you need to be their advocate. And you need to do it at lightning speed.

And then there's the hypervigilance. Determined to be in control of our lives, to be at home and out of hospital, parents are prepared to take on a huge responsibility of care. You don't even realise at the time. I know I didn't, looking back – how the hell did I get to the point where I was running the equivalent of a high-dependency unit at home?

I was charged with keeping my child alive. Making decisions, administering drugs and therapies and carrying out procedures that if done incorrectly would be fatal. I had to stay focused and on it.

I lived with the constant feeling that if I fell apart, then everything would fall apart. As parents, our antennae are up all the time. We see the subtleties in our child's condition, and our instincts guide us. And that all takes its toll.

We worry about making a mistake that could kill our child. We worry about making the wrong decision. We worry about leaving our child with other people. We worry about our other children. There is no respite from the worry. It's no wonder many parents mentioned PTSD when I spoke to them.

Parents of children with complex medical needs have to become experts on their child. This world is so far removed from the world of 'normal' parenting. Slowly, and before you even realise it's happened, you find yourself spouting the medical jargon, discussing fluid balances, interpreting blood test results, reeling off the names of drugs. You become adept at performing medical procedures – sometimes you are the only one trained on the hospital ward at that point in time.

It's a 24/7 life, but one where, over and over, parents told me that they struggled to have their role and contribution valued, their voices heard.

What needs to change? What can professionals working to support families caring for a child with complex needs take from this book?

During my conversations with parents and family members, with other professionals and through my own lived experience I have found that it boils down to three things.

How would you feel if it was you?

If you are a professional working with families caring for a child with complex needs, please understand that this is really bloody hard for us. You may not like the parent sitting opposite you, but please empathise and understand where they've come from to get here.

Empathy. Very different from sympathy. It's about listening and acknowledging, allowing yourself to enter our space and feel a little of what it's like for us. It's about walking beside us but not judging us. Sympathy, on the other hand, means understanding someone else's suffering. It's more cognitive in nature and keeps a certain distance.

Take off your metaphorical white coat and be a human interacting with another human. Just like Kate Granger, the founder of the #HelloMyNameIs campaign, you never know when the tables could be turned.

Never forget that your words have an impact. Parents hang on what you say and how you say it. What may be a throwaway comment for you can feel like life and death for a parent.

My friend Renata sums it up: 'Kindness will always be the most important thing you bring to the room. Never forget it, no matter how tired or stressed or important you become.'

Don't call me Mum!

I can't emphasise this enough. This isn't about titles; it's about enabling parents to know and feel that their contribution is valued. It's about humanising your interactions with them. So the starting point is getting to know us as people. Stepping into our space. Understanding the role we play in keeping our child alive, 24/7, when you go home, when you go on holiday, when you are off duty. We don't get to switch off, ever.

I have learned that some parents don't mind being called Mum or Dad, and that's fine. But what they universally do mind is not having their contribution acknowledged. Feeling that they are just an item on the agenda. Parents need to feel valued, and this means having a seat at the table. Asking someone what they want to be called is the first step in humanising the interaction, telling the parent, 'I see you.'

Remember, these are parents who are embedded in the system. Not occasional visitors to it. Think how it must feel if a parent has been living on an inpatient ward with their child for weeks at a time, and nobody has bothered to learn their name? Can you imagine how depersonalising that feels? Especially when they are the ones who know the minutiae about their child's care and how to manage it?

Most parents will be forgiving of the busy staff member who has just come on shift and met them for the first time. They will be less forgiving if they are sitting in a multi-disciplinary meeting with a group of professionals, and they are referred to as 'Mum' or 'Dad' when everyone else around the table is called by their name or an agreed title.

I was not just 'Mum'. I craved the opportunity to *just* be Daisy's mum. Instead, I was her nurse, her teacher, her carer, her advocate, her housekeeper, her driver, her translator. I was all the things that parents of medically complex children have to take on to keep their child safe and well. I was an extreme parent.

Respect the role we play in keeping our child alive and the lack of support we have to be able to do this. The risks we are prepared to take on, which professionals know would never be accepted anywhere else. Working a double shift? Administering a controlled drug without another staff member checking the dose? Juggling our child's care with caring for other children, who may also have their own unique needs?

That's the essence of 'Don't call me Mum'. Give parents of medically complex children the respect and understanding they deserve for what they do and the sacrifices they make to keep their child alive.

It's OK to say you don't know

I go back to those moments when professionals were honest with me. When they spoke about 'academic guesswork' or not knowing what was going on with Daisy. Far from being disappointed or upset, I was actually reassured by this. At least we knew what we were dealing with, that we didn't have false hope. And it fostered a spirit of collaboration to work together to find out what was wrong.

This feeling was echoed in the conversations I had with parents I interviewed for this book.

As Gemma told me, 'Don't fob me off; I know what you're doing. Just tell me you don't know.'

Our Western medicine approach is focused on fixing things. We hear the good news stories about children being cured. Healthcare charities rely on these stories to generate income, after all. No wonder we're shocked and upset when children can't be fixed. When children die.

The reality is that doctors can't always fix things. They don't always have the answers. Sometimes a child remains undiagnosed. And we need to change our culture to make this acceptable. To accept that sometimes children die.

Saying 'I don't know' is a step towards showing that we are all human, trying to do the best we can. And it's a way of opening up more collaborative conversations. It moves the narrative from false hope to realistic expectations. The way we talk about prognosis is one example. Do we really know how a patient will respond to treatment? What works for one may not work for another.

How realistically can a doctor say, 'This treatment has a 10 per cent chance of working'? How do they know that? Where does that figure come from? Parents will hang on to these figures, the prognosis, but do we really know how each child will respond to treatment, to a therapy?

I was told that Daisy would only live for a year, yet she lived for 12. Natalie was told that children with her son Louie's condition did not survive past the age of three, yet he died when he was seven.

The more we understand human genetics, and the more break-throughs that are made around treatments and cures, the less we should be reliant on generalised statistics and prognosis. Healthcare is becoming increasingly personalised to an individual, so shouldn't this mean we need to move away from general sweeping assumptions of prognosis and chances of success?

Maybe this approach will help reframe the narrative of win or lose, so that we can begin to have open and honest conversations around death and dying. So that introducing palliative care is not seen as giving up on the child. So that professionals, regardless of their speciality, understand what palliative care can bring and make it part of the conversation.

Daisy was supported by palliative services for many years. She was not actively dying; she was actively living. In the end, no one really knew how long she would live, but thanks to early referrals to palliative services, we were able to maintain the best quality of life possible for her until the last few months of her life.

Start those difficult conversations early. Be brave and know that to say 'I don't know' does not make you a failure. It makes you human.

These three things – 'How would you feel if it was you?', 'Don't call me Mum!' and 'It's OK to say you don't know' – are all about communication. About how we interact with each other.

So why are we not teaching this in medical school? On nursing degrees? Why is communication seen as a 'soft skill' that you can go on a course to learn and gain continuing professional development credits?

It should be at the heart of how we train people who have chosen to work in a health and social care profession. This is a people profession, and it involves communicating with people at their most vulnerable. This can't be taught during a two-day professional skills course. It needs to be embedded, part of the culture. Many nurses and doctors have told me that they learned how to communicate well from observing the very best and the very worst examples in their day-to-day work.

Parents of medically complex children don't have time for the professionals to catch up. They need to feel listened to, empathised with and understood. Get it right, listen actively and ensure that a parent's contribution is valued. That's when good communication and collaboration happens.

It involves a culture shift. Creating a better balance between a patriarchal medicine approach of 'doctor knows best' and one where parents feel abandoned to autonomy. It's about meeting in the middle and respecting what each party brings to the table.

Because communication is a two-way street.

Andy, my late husband, was trained in neuro-linguistic programming. He used these techniques to help his clients improve their communications within the workplace. One of the most important lessons he shared was that the only thing you have control over, when trying to change how others relate to you, is to change yourself and how you relate to them.

This is what I want parents to know. Think about the impact of your own communication style and the response it elicits.

Our world is about fighting for things, and it's so easy to slip into the language of combat, setting up the potential for conflict. I wanted the teams on my side. I needed them to be on my side, and I needed them to hear me and know me. I needed to know that Daisy's needs were their priority.

I worked hard to ensure that, in meetings and appointments, the professionals on the other side of the bed or desk got to know Daisy as a little girl, not just a patient. I would try to be assertive without falling into aggression (easier said than done when you're mentally and physically exhausted). I would try to just be nice, even if I didn't like the consultant. Ultimately, conflict and breakdown in communication doesn't help, it doesn't move things forward and it doesn't help the most important person at the centre. The child.

Parents, please don't do it on your own. I spend a lot of time these days working with parents as an advocate and supporter. Attending meetings with them, writing letters, going to outpatient's appointments. I struggled on my own for many years. I now sit in meetings with other parents, and I look back and wish I'd asked for help. I wished I'd asked people to just come to the meetings, speak on my behalf when I was so broken and exhausted from fighting. To have someone (who was not emotionally involved) to speak to without judgement, to be a sounding board and supporter.

Advocacy. Someone to help me speak. How valuable would that have been? Especially in the early days. There's an element of it in the work of chaplaincy services in hospitals, but I always thought chaplains were for people of faith. I was so wrong. We need better access to impartial and independent advocacy support for parents who are stumbling around in this complicated, highly charged and emotional world to help them adjust and adapt, and for their voices to be heard.

And if things do start to break down, we need better access to mediation services so that both parties – parents as well as professionals – can share their feelings and hopefully come to a resolution.

Mediation can be a game-changer in building trust and understanding between parents and professionals. As this comment from a parent who was involved in mediation illustrates:

> The first meeting was an eye-opener to how both sides were feeling. It was just like giving us space for both teams to walk towards something, towards a goal together, not like walking from different perspectives.

It works both ways. Here's feedback from a nurse who was involved in mediation with a family:

It absolutely changed how we felt...it made me realise that this is a set of parents that are absolutely, desperately wanting the best for their baby... It made us think, it made us reflect and see where we had, not gone wrong, but where communication could have been much, much better.[1]

Mediation and advocacy, when used properly and at the right time, are essential elements in improving how medical professionals and parents communicate and collaborate. The final piece of this jigsaw is the need for a more formalised ethics process that understands that it's not just there for the clinicians but for the parents, too. This means allowing parents an opportunity to present their own viewpoint to the committee rather than via the lens of their clinician. We need to revisit the arbitrary and informal arrangements for clinical ethics committees and consider whether parent/carer representation should always be part of that forum.

Looking back at my time as the parent of a child with medical complexity, I think I got a lot of things right, but that was more by luck than judgement. We had some great professionals who were prepared to go above and beyond. I worked hard to make the system work. I wrote emails and letters and tried to use social media in a positive way. I was just acutely aware that I needed people on my side to ensure I got the best for Daisy.

Things did go wrong. I had an unsubstantiated complaint made about my behaviour to social services. Thankfully, the professionals who knew me and my situation were on the case immediately to provide evidence that the claim was unfounded and ethically wrong. In hindsight, I shudder at the thought of what would have happened if I didn't have those relationships with the professionals. If I had had to fight to be believed.

The most important lesson I have learned in reflecting back on my time caring for Daisy is that I lost myself. I lost who I was as I

---

1   Thank you to the Medical Mediation Foundation for gaining permission from both respondents and allowing me to share both these quotes.

became Daisy's mum. And it's taken me all this time to reclaim my own identity as separate from my child's.

That would be the one most important piece of advice for any parent caring for a medically complex child. Remember who you are. Don't lose sight of yourself. One day, you will have to find that person again. You will have changed and grown and be scarred and battered by your experience, but the essence of who you were will still be there. Don't lose them.

Daisy taught me to live in the moment. To take one day at a time. To unbuckle my seatbelt and enjoy the ride.

If I was an outsider looking into my life at that time, I would have assumed it was sad and tragic. But it was so far from that. There was so much laughter and joy. And nothing was ever taken for granted. The little things in life were appreciated as big things. There is nothing more liberating than knowing your time together is finite; you choose how you are going to spend that time carefully.

In our family, we talk about death openly and freely. We knew from day one that the clock was ticking with Daisy and, ironically, that attitude helped us cope with the shock of Andy's terminal diagnosis. Daisy taught us how to live. And that's what we wanted from the professionals around us. The understanding and support to get on with our finite lives with Daisy. Not having to fight for care packages or shout to make our voices heard.

There is a huge, empty void in my life now that Daisy is no longer here. I would give anything for one last cuddle, to hear her call out 'Mummy', to ruffle her funny curly hair. I miss her desperately. The grief is visceral. But I would not want her back. Not with the pain and deterioration that she experienced in her final months. I take huge comfort from knowing that, at the end of Daisy's life, I knew it was time to say goodbye. It was time to do the most selfless thing a parent could do and let my child go.

I did the right thing for Daisy, even though it didn't feel like the right thing for me at the time. And in doing so, I knew that, despite the enormous anguish I would always feel, I was doing anything for my child.